MALARIA & POVERTY IN AFRICA

MALARIA & POVERTY IN AFRICA

Edited by
Augustin Kwasi Fosu
Germano Mwabu

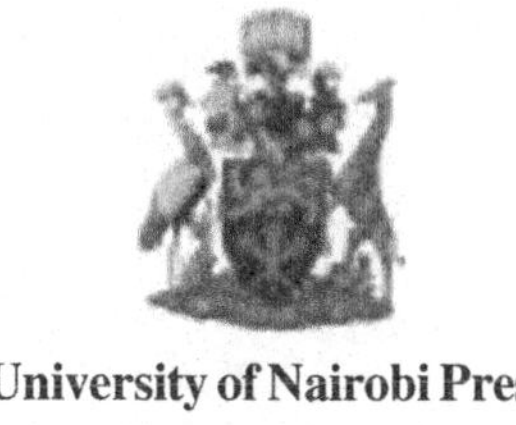

University of Nairobi Press

First published 2007 by
University of Nairobi Press (UONP)
Jomo Kenyatta Memorial Library
University of Nairobi
P.O. Box 30197 – 00100 Nairobi
E-mail: nup@uonbi.ac.ke
www.uonbi.ac.ke/press

The University of Nairobi Press supports and promotes University of Nairobi's objectives of discovery, dissemination and preservation of knowledge, and stimulation of intellectual and cultural life by publishing works of the highest quality in association with partners in different parts of the world. In doing so, it adheres to the University's tradition of excellence, innovation and scholarship.

University of Nairobi Library Cataloging-in Publication Data
Malaria and Poverty in Africa / ed by A.K. Fosu and G. Mwabu:– Nairobi: University of Nairobi Press, 2007 pp. 199.
1. Malaria. 2. Poverty. I. Title, II Fosu, Augustin Kwasi, III Mwabu, Germano.
RA 644.M3 M2.

ISBN 978-9966-846-63-1

The University of Nairobi Press wishes to acknowledge permission by the Kenyan Ministry of Health to use, with slight adaptation, the "Stop Malaria Save a Life" logo on the cover.

Printed by
English Press Ltd
Nairobi.

Table of Contents

List of Tables, Figures and Appendices

Tables

Figures

Chapter Appendices

Foreword

Malaria has persisted in Africa for decades despite national and multilateral efforts to control the disease. The disease has severely retarded economic and social development in the region. According to some estimates, malaria-prone regions have per capita incomes several times lower than malaria-free countries.

The chapters in this volume analyze the nexus between poverty and malaria, with a focus on policies that can be implemented at different levels of society to fight the disease. The book begins with an explanation of the nature of the poverty and malaria relationships, and identifies approaches to meeting the many challenges posed by the epidemic. The volume is an outcome of a collaborative research project on malaria and poverty in Africa sponsored by the African Economic Research Consortium (AERC).

The African Economic Research Consortium strengthens local capacity for conducting independent, rigorous inquiry into problems facing the management of the economies in sub-Saharan Africa via learning by doing, and supports postgraduate training in economics through collaborative masters and PhD programs. It is the foremost institution in the promotion of policy-relevant research on poverty in Africa.

The research findings reported in this volume should be highly valuable in the design of programs to fight malaria and poverty in Africa and elsewhere. I strongly recommend this book to anyone interested in understanding the connections between poverty and malaria, as well as the policies that can be implemented to control malaria and encourage growth and development in Sub-Saharan Africa.

William Lyakurwa
Executive Director, AERC
Nairobi, Kenya.

Preface

Malaria is a serious health and economic problem in Africa, afflicting more than half of the continent's population. The disease kills nearly one million children in Sub-Saharan Africa each year, with several million more in their prime working age unable to perform to their potential due to regular bouts of malaria. It has severely retarded economic development in many countries in the region, with poverty and isolation being some of its most visible consequences. Although HIV/AIDS, tuberculosis, and nutritional deficiencies also pose major development problems on the continent, the challenges presented by malaria are of a different kind, because the disease is widespread, persistent, and grossly underestimated by the general population. The importance of malaria, along with HIV/AIDS and other diseases in the development agenda, is now recognized in Goal 6 of the Millennium Development Goals (MDGs).

Unlike HIV/AIDS, malaria is currently without stigma, despite its deadly nature, and ordinary citizens believe that its cure is widely available and accessible, a belief that was to some extent warranted before malaria became resistant to chloroquine. The new anti-malarial drugs, the Artemisinin-based Combination Therapies (ACTs), are not as widely available as the previous first-line drugs. And the cost of their recommended dosage for a bout of malaria is more than twice the international poverty line of $1.00 per day, so that the dose is not affordable by the vast majority of the African population. An annual subsidy of US $300–500 million, has recently been recommended to the international community by the Institute of Medicine of the USA National Academies of Science (Kenneth Arrow, Hellen Gelband and Claire Panosian, 2004, *Saving Lives, Buying Time: Economics of Malaria Drugs in an Age of Resistance,* National Academies Press, Washington, D.C), to help bring down the prices of ACTs to the prevailing level of the cost of chloroquine dosage. If implemented, the subsidy would make the new drugs widely affordable. Even so, their usage in remote villages and in urban slums in Africa could severely be limited by inefficient drug distribution systems, as well as by ineffective health care-seeking behaviors of the population.

Attempts to control malaria in Africa have encountered several major difficulties. First, information has been lacking on the magnitudes of the economic and social burdens of the disease, information that is needed to motivate policy makers to design and implement control programs. Second, little information has been available about the economic behavior of households in seeking treatment for malaria or in finding ways to avoid the disease. Thus, incentives for encouraging households to engage in malaria control strategies could not be properly designed or implemented. Third, in many African countries, little is known about drug distribution systems in private or public sectors through which malaria control products and services are delivered to populations. Consequently, information for reforming these systems to make them more effective has been lacking.

The chapters in this volume are designed to help rectify the above situations. The book begins with an explanation of the nature of the poverty and malaria problem, and identifies possible approaches to meeting the challenge. The approaches are based on country case studies designed to reflect the various sub-regions of the African sub-continent. The remainder of the volume provides important information for designing specific malaria control programs, and for reforming national drug distribution systems.

We are grateful to the authors of the chapters for effectively contributing to this volume, and to the African Economic Research Consortium (AERC) secretariat for the very valuable financial and logistical support. We thank Prof. Erik Thorbecke for conceptualizing the poverty project, under whose auspices this work was carried out and for successfuly launching the project jointly with Prof. Ali G. Ali.

Augustin Fosu and Germano Mwabu

March, 2007

List of Contributors

Augustin Kwasi Fosu, United Nations Economic Commission for Africa (UNECA), Addis Ababa, Ethiopia.

Germano Mwabu, University of Nairobi, Nairobi, Kenya.

Flora Musonda, Economic and Social Research Foundation, Dar es Salaam, Tanzania.

Francis Mangani, University of Zambia, Lusaka, Zambia.

Bernadette Dia Kamgnia, University of Yaounde II, Yaounde, Cameroon.

Olufunke A. Olagoke, University of Ibadan, Ibadan, Nigeria.

Part I

Background

Chapter 1

Introduction

Augustin Kwasi Fosu and Germano Mwabu

Malaria is a serious problem in Africa. It afflicts more than one-half of the continent's population. The disease kills nearly one million children in Sub-Saharan Africa (SSA) each year, with several million more in their prime working age unable to perform to their potential due to regular bouts of malaria. It has severely retarded economic development in many countries in the region. The importance of malaria, along with HIV/AIDS and other diseases in the development agenda, is now recognized in Goal 6 of the Millennium Development Goals (MDGs).

Malaria also has major adverse implications for poverty, which in turn affects about one-half of the African population. If we are to achieve Goal 1 of the MDGs of halving poverty by 2015, then the malaria challenge must be met head on. Attempts to control the disease on the sub-continent so far have failed for several reasons. First, there has been lack of information on the magnitude of the economic and social burden of the disease, information that would have motivated policy makers to design and implement more effective control programs. Second, little is known about the economic behavior of households in seeking treatment or prevention for malaria, thus making it difficult to design appropriate policy incentives for households to effectively allocate resources toward malaria control. Third, in many African countries, there is little knowledge about drug distribution systems in private or public sectors through which anti-malaria drugs, as well as other malaria control products and services, are delivered to populations. Consequently, these systems cannot be properly reformed for effective delivery of anti-malarials.

The chapters in this volume are designed to address the above gaps. The volume begins by shedding light on the nature of the poverty and malaria problem. It then provides information that can be used to design malaria control strategies and to reform existing programs in order to reflect new malaria realities on the sub-continent, particularly the new strains of drug resistant malaria. The role of insecticide-treated bed nets in controlling malaria is also examined.

Part one of the book comprises two chapters, including this introduction. Part 2 contains four case studies from four countries, namely, Cameroon, Kenya, Nigeria, and Zambia. These case studies are designed to reflect the realities of the four sub-regions of SSA.

The second chapter of part one, by Germano Mwabu and Augustin Kwasi Fosu, sets the stage for case studies by articulating the critical issues in malaria and poverty in Africa. Some of the issues analyzed include the state of malaria in Africa; a historical account of global malaria control and eradication efforts; the inter-relationship between malaria and poverty: how malaria affects poverty, via growth for instance, and vice-versa; economic benefits and costs of malaria control; and a range of economic and social factors that should be taken into account in the design of malaria control programs.

Mwabu and Fosu find that the economic toll of malaria in Africa amounts to at least ten percent of gross domestic product per year. Moreover, the cumulative effects of malaria are enormous. For example, per capita GDP of malaria-endemic countries in tropical Africa in the 1990s was only one-third of GDP of countries that had been free of malaria three decades earlier in the 1960s (Gallup and Sachs, 2000). Mwabu and Fosu argue that the debate should now shift from malaria eradication to control, for the objective of malaria eradication, which was thought to be achievable in the 1940s and 1950s, is now believed to be unattainable. Thus, an appropriate cost-benefit analysis is required to determine the level and nature of malaria control programs. Furthermore, a proper measurement of the economic benefits of a malaria control program requires that the effects of other intervening factors on malaria reduction be isolated. Identifying such factors and disentangling their effects in turn require generating additional information that can be used to design malaria control programs and measure their economic effects.

Part two of the volume presents four country case studies drawn from different parts of SSA: East, West, Central and Southern Africa, respectively. Chapter three by Germano Mwabu, is the first of these studies. It examines the economic burden of malaria in Kenya. Mwabu reviews existing studies and shows that seventy per cent of the Kenyan population suffers from malaria infection at one point or another during the year. Malaria prevalence in Kenya is highest in Western, Nyanza and Coast provinces, and has remained quite stable in these regions for many decades, suggesting the need for geographical targeting of anti-malaria interventions. Malaria in Kenya is resistant to chloroquine, a drug that is no longer officially used in the first line of malaria treatment in the country. However, its unauthorized use appears widespread, a situation that could increase malaria prevalence in a population where, already, over 50 per cent of outpatient visits are malaria-related (Republic of Kenya, 1996).

Using household data for 1994, Mwabu shows that malaria morbidity in Kenya is associated with a 15–16 per cent reduction in wage incomes, with a 10–21 per cent decline in farm output during the long rains, and with a much higher reduction in household income. These economic burdens of malaria are generally of the same orders of magnitude as those reported in the macro-econometric literature. The chapter shows that farm output is relatively elastic with respect to disease prevalence and that the economic burden of malaria is greater than the burden for other illnesses. In particular, a ten per cent increase in malaria prevalence reduces farm output by three percent, compared with a 1.3 per cent output reduction associated with other diseases. The last part of the chapter is devoted to a discussion of how the chapter's findings can be applied to the design and implementation of effective malaria control programs.

In chapter four, Olufunke Olagoke examines the economic burden of childhood malaria in Nigeria. This chapter is a welcome differentiation from the Kenyan study, which investigates malaria burden within the whole population. Beginning with the Nigerian population as a whole, however, Olagoke reports that between 1980 and 1996, malaria mortality and morbidity increased as poverty in the country worsened. She stresses that there is a strong association between malaria and poverty in Nigeria. Because malaria is a major reason for outpatient visits and hospital admissions in Nigeria, households spend large sums of money on malaria treatment and prevention.

Olagoke reports further that households can spend up to US$ 25 per month on malaria treatments and nearly thirteen per cent of monthly farm income on malaria prevention activities.

Olagoke then delves into the main subject of the chapter: "direct" and "indirect" costs of malaria in children. Direct costs are the out-of-pocket expenses of treating and preventing a malaria episode, including travel, accommodation and related expenses incurred by persons seeking treatment on behalf of the child. Indirect costs comprise the opportunity cost of the time used to seek treatment for the child and the child's loss of school time.

Olagoke finds that the average total cost of an episode of malaria for a Nigerian child is around US$ 44.34; however, the cost varies by employment status of the caregiver, who is typically the mother. The cost is US $44 for the self-employed, US$ 35 for the government employee and US $27.50 for the unemployed caregiver. This cost also varies by gender of the caregiver and by his/her education attainment. At ninety per cent, the share of the indirect component represents the lion's share of the total cost.

The author finds that ninety per cent of the malaria cases are managed at home and that most caregivers associate malaria with mosquito bites. However, although nearly fifty per cent of households use mosquito nets to prevent malarial illnesses, they are unaware that insecticide-treated bed nets are a relatively effective means of malaria prevention, suggesting that health education can be an important strategy for malaria control. The chapter ends with detailed recommendations of interventions for improving home-based management of childhood malaria, and for increasing treatment efficacy at health facilities.

The fifth chapter, by Bernadette Kamgnia, briefly reviews the malaria situation in Cameroon and presents a detailed analysis of demand for malaria treatment and prevention services in an urban community of Yaounde. Kamgnia reports that thirty to fifty per cent of medical consultations in Cameroon are for malaria treatment, and that twenty five to forty five per cent of deaths among children are due to malaria. Apart from its toll on health, malaria's economic burden is also large; malaria accounts for nearly seventy five per cent of the days of work lost due to illness, and for about forty per cent of the annual household health expenditure. The disease is of great concern at all levels of the health care system in Cameroon, because it is resistant to some of the drugs, notably chloroquine, which is one of the most commonly used drugs in the treatment of malaria.

As in other countries, the malaria control program in Cameroon is based on a combination of malaria treatment and prevention activities. Kamgnia examines the demand for services and products of these activities, focusing on how that demand is affected by households' knowledge about the cause and transmission of malaria. Using survey data that she collected from an urban community in Cameroon in 2001, Kamgnia finds that ninety nine percent of households in Yaounde were aware of malaria as a disease at the time of the survey. Furthermore, eighty per cent of the households associated malaria with mosquito bites. However, only a small proportion of households (5.2%) knew that malaria could be prevented by insecticide-treated bed nets; again pointing to the importance of education in malaria control.

While the Ministry of Public Health is the main source of insecticide-treated bed nets in Yaounde, it is not the principal source of malaria treatment. About forty seven per cent of malaria patients relied on self-care, while forty one per cent sought treatment from modern health facilities, including government clinics; and ten per cent from traditional healers. Quinine was the most commonly used anti-malarial drug. Other medications were antipyretics, chloroquine, amodiaquine, P-sulfadioxine and artemisinin.

It emerges from Kamgnia's study that the main determinants of the demand for malaria treatment include the availability of anti-malarial drugs, the cost of treatment, and socioeconomic characteristics of patients such as education, sex, and age. In particular, the cost of care at health facilities reduces the demand for malaria treatment, as does the non-availability of anti-malarial drugs. Education increases the utilization of modern health facilities for malaria treatment and reduces the probability of utilizing anti-malarial drugs of uncertain quality.

Generally, informal sources of anti-malarial drugs tend to be patronized by persons with low levels of schooling. Since poverty is strongly correlated with low educational achievement (see Republic of Kenya, 1996, for the case of Kenya, East Africa, for example), Kamgnia's study suggests that the poor are at greater risk of receiving ineffective anti-malarial treatment compared with the non-poor. Thus concerns for the plight of the poor require that policies be designed to improve the quality of informal anti-malarial medications.

In the sixth and final chapter, Flora Musonda and Francis Mangani examine the issue of pharmaceutical supplies in relation to national malaria control efforts, using Zambia as a case study. The authors show that malaria is endemic in Zambia, and up to twenty per cent of the mortality in the country is attributable to the disease. Since 1976, malaria prevalence increased rapidly from 122 cases per thousand to nearly 400 cases per thousand in 1998.

The chapter identifies six main sources of drugs and pharmaceutical supplies for the health facilities in the country: private retail and wholesale distribution system, the local drug manufacturers, the Ministry of Health, the non-government organizations, donors, and the Medical Stores Limited. Most of the pharmaceutical products used in the country are imported. The Ministry of Health is the largest importer, accounting for forty six per cent of the value of drug imports in 1996. The wholesalers sell drugs at a profit to commercial pharmacies and to health facilities.

The Medical Stores Ltd., which has a special role in the area of pharmaceutical drugs, is an example of an organization that both imports and distributes drugs directly to the retailers. It serves as the government's storage and distribution agent, and is responsible for distributing to individual health facilities drugs procured directly by the Ministry of Health. In addition, it distributes essential drug kits financed by donors to all health centers in the country at a fee.

Despite the elaborate drug distribution system, Musonda and Mangani report that the government health facilities experience frequent shortages of anti-malarial drugs. These shortages are partly blamed for the emergence of drug-resistant malaria in Zambia. In particular, the shortages have been associated with sub-optimal treatment of malaria using chloroquine, which in 1990s was still the drug of choice in Zambia, as in other countries in Africa, for the first line of malaria treatment. The chloroquine failure rate is fifty two per cent, which means that only about half of the malaria patients treated with chloroquine recover. Alternative anti-malarial drugs in the country, and less commonly used, include fansidar, quinine, artemisinin and halfantin.

Musonda and Mangani argue that the main factors contributing to drug-resistant malaria in Zambia include: over-use of chloroquine mainly due to self-prescription behavior of patients; outdated malaria prevention methods; high costs of insecticide-treated nets; introduction of cost-sharing in public health facilities; and the lack of malaria diagnostic equipment in government health facilities.

As a strategy for effectively combating malaria in Zambia, the authors recommend a modification in drug policies, emphasizing discontinuation of chloroquine as the first line of treatment, given its high failure rate. The authors argue that switching to other drugs is feasible because alternative anti-malarial drugs are available, and are acceptable to the government and the general population.

References

Gallup, J.L. and Sachs, J.D.(2000), "The Economic Burden of Malaria", Harvard University, Center for International Development, CID Working Paper No. 52, July.

Kamgnia, B. (2007), "The Demand for Malaria Control Products and Services: Evidence from Yaounde, Cameroon", this Volume.

Musonda, F.M. and Mangani, F. (2007), "The Distribution of Pharmaceutical Products and Malaria Control in Zambia", this Volume.

Mwabu, G. (2007), "The Economic Burden of Malaria in Kenya", this volume.

Mwabu, G. and Fosu, A.K. (2007), "Understanding Malaria and Poverty in Africa: A Framework", this Volume.

Olagoke, A.O. (2007), "The Economic Burden of Childhood Malaria in Nigeria", this Volume.

Kenya, Republic of (1996), *Welfare Monitoring Survey: Basic Report, 1994*. Nairobi: Ministry of Planning and National Development.

Chapter 2

Understanding Malaria and Poverty in Africa: A Framework

Germano Mwabu and Augustin Kwasi Fosu

2.0 Introduction

Poverty and malaria are widespread in Africa. Over fifty per cent of the African people are poor, and most of them are afflicted more by malaria than by any other disease in their lifetime. The simultaneous occurrence of poverty and malaria in much of Sub-Saharan Africa is not accidental. These self-reinforcing facets of underdevelopment in Africa seem to have the same underlying causes. Alleviation of poverty and control of malaria require that these common underlying causes be identified, understood, and effectively addressed by public policy. The control of malaria would reduce the spread, depth and severity of poverty, and poverty reduction in turn would facilitate malaria control. Throughout this chapter, therefore, the terms "poverty reduction" and "malaria control" are used instead of the term eradication. Eradication of poverty and malaria should be viewed as long-term goals, with reduction and control being intermediate goals.

Malaria is a serious problem in Africa by any standard (see Olagoke, this volume). Even when account is taken of the HIV/AIDS pandemic, malaria still remains an important source of morbidity in Sub-Saharan Africa. The large disease burden from malaria in Africa is evidenced by high intensity of malaria bites, which average around 200–300 per person per year. At least 300–500 million malaria episodes are treated annually in Sub-Saharan Africa (American Association for the Advancement of Science, 1991). The disease afflicts mainly pregnant women, young children, migratory populations and persons with little previous exposure to malaria attack (Snow, *et al.*, 1999).

2.1 Economic Burden of Malaria

Apart from the pathogenic burden just noted, the economic burden from malaria is also immense. Malaria adversely affects economic growth, and is thus one of the main factors responsible for the persistence of poverty in Sub-Saharan Africa. The annual loss of GDP per capita from malaria is estimated at 1.3 per cent per year. In Africa, where malaria is present all year round, this annual erosion of economic growth would reduce gross domestic product by nearly 20 twenty per cent over a fifteen year period (African Summit on Roll Back Malaria, April 25, 2000).

Apart from easily measurable human and economic costs of malaria, there are many costs that are not reflected in the total burden of malaria because they are hard to measure. To start with, the cost of the pain and suffering inflicted by malaria episodes and deaths is excluded from the cost burden of malaria. Yet people are willing to pay several times the direct loss of income caused by malaria to avoid the pain, anxiety and uncertainty associated with the disease (African Summit on Roll Back Malaria, 2000).

The calculation of the cost burden of malaria often concentrates on short-run costs such as labor time loss due to malaria, costs of malaria treatment and prevention, and productivity losses caused by premature deaths. Ignored in such calculations are long-term costs such as losses in human capital formation arising from the disruption of children's learning by malaria sicknesses; and productivity losses due to inefficient long-run settlement patterns of the population.

Even though the human and economic costs of malaria may seem intuitively obvious, it is extremely difficult to empirically demonstrate their magnitude at the household level. Self-reporting of malaria morbidity, for example, tends to understate the malaria problem among the poor and the less educated, as these sub-populations generally report the disease only when it is at advanced stages. Furthermore, clinical diagnosis of the problem in the community on a large scale is extremely expensive and is rarely done. It is even more difficult to show a connection between labor productivity losses and malaria morbidity because of the substitution of tasks within households in the event of a malarial episode, which reduces or averts altogether the impact of the disease on production. Farm households in malarious areas also tend to plant crops which are little affected by labor time losses due to malaria (Conly, 1975; Herrin and Rosenfield, 1988). However, comparable firm-level evidence of malaria on industrial production is lacking. Thus, although at the macro-level econometric studies show large statistical losses of national wealth from malaria, studies at the micro-level often find no such effects of malaria.

Given that malaria is widespread in Africa, and its toll on human life and welfare is large, we start from a testable presumption that malaria is an important determinant of poverty. However, poverty being a multidimensional phenomenon, it remains to be investigated as to what dimensions of it are due to malaria. As noted above, income poverty may not be statistically associated with malaria incidence at the household level. This lack of statistical relationship is not least due to the complexity of the association between malaria and poverty. Because of its intricate nature, the relationship may not be detectable with cross-sectional data or with data obtained from certain survey designs. In this regard, it should be recognized that poverty is a cause as well as a consequence of malaria. Poverty predisposes individuals to malaria, and malaria in turn reduces incomes of individuals, thus further eroding their ability to afford malaria treatments and prevention. These intricate issues are explored in detail in a later section.

Malarial deaths and morbidity in Africa vary greatly from one region to another because of the differences in malaria transmission mechanisms, which include cultural, economic, environmental, and political factors. These factors vary substantially even within neighboring villages. Thus, no single factor can be pinpointed as the primary cause of malaria. Consequently, interventions for malaria control should be region and context specific.

2.2 Malaria Control and Eradication

The control and eventual eradication of malaria in Africa is a complex problem involving a combination of medical, bio-environmental, economic and other approaches (see Sharma *et al.*, 1991). The problem can start to be addressed in African villages through the application of biomedical technology and cost-effective management of control programs; mediated by efficient responses to malaria episodes by individuals, households, and communities. This integrative approach assigns equal importance to supply and demand-side factors in the control of malaria, as well as to institutional arrangements through which governments, non-governmental organizations and communities would interact in that endeavor.

Key to the success of such an approach is information about malaria (transmission, prevalence and strain) and the available control methods, including their costs and effectiveness. Also critical in the design of effective control programs is information about control measures already being undertaken by households and communities as well as the control measures preferred by households and individuals.

This chapter has six sections following this introduction. In section two, a brief description of malaria transmission mechanisms are described. In section three, we provide a historical account of malaria control and eradication programs since the early 1950s. Conceptual issues in the nexus between malaria and poverty are pursued in section four, where epidemiological principles of malaria control are also discussed. In section five, we return to the issue of malaria burden highlighted in the introduction, and present a detailed account of malaria risks, and mortality among children in Africa. Economic studies on malaria in Africa are briefly reviewed in section six, with a focus on cost-effectiveness studies. In section seven, we highlight knowledge gaps in malaria control, and suggest possible research topics to close these gaps.

2.3 Transmission of Malaria

2.3.1 African malaria vectors and parasites

Malaria vectors are invertebrate species carrying protozoan parasites that cause malaria sickness in people. While a detailed account of the etiology of human malaria is outside the scope of this chapter (see Bruce-Chwatt, 1986), it should be noted that malaria infection and disease occur only when malaria parasites are transmitted from its host, that is, an infected mosquito vector to the blood stream of a human being via a mosquito bite. Without such a simple transmission, malaria cannot occur in humans. The difficulty, however, is that for numerous reasons the transmission is extremely difficult to prevent (see Snow *et al.*, 1999).

In Africa, there are four main malaria vectors: *Anopheles gambiae* (a complex of six species), *Anopheles funestes*, *Anopheles pharoensis* and *Anopheles arabiensis*, the last of which is dominant in the Sudan. In contrast, the main malaria vectors in other world regions, especially in India, include *Anopheles fluviatilis*, *Anopheles minimus* and *Anopheles culicifacies* (Sharma *et al.*, 1991).

In Africa, female Anopheles mosquitoes have shown resistance to numerous insecticides; are widely distributed; and inflict high rates of inoculations in humans in a wide range of geographic, seasonal and ecological conditions (Coluzzi, 1984; as cited in American Association for the Advancement of Science, 1991).

Information on methods of dealing with these vectors (e.g., bed nets, repellants, window screens, community-based anti-malaria public works, etc), including costs and efficacy of the methods, is important in the design of effective control strategies. Specifically, knowledge of supply of, and demand for malaria control devices and services in specific locations and communities is critical for efficient implementation of control programs.

The four malaria parasites that are transmitted by the above variety of vectors are *Plasmodium falciparum* (which accounts for the most severe cases of malaria and for over ninety per cent of malaria infections in Tropical Africa); *P. vivax*, *P. malariae*, and *P. ovale* (see Bruce-Chwatt, 1986). Some of these parasites are increasingly becoming resistant to common anti-malaria drugs in many parts of Africa.

For example, *P. falciparum* is known to have been resistant to chloroquine in East Africa since the 1970s. In Kenya, the first case of chloroquine resistant *P. falciparum* was reported among Kenyan infants in 1982. After this date, the resistance spread rapidly and in early 2000, the Kenyan Ministry of Health stopped the use of chloroquine in the treatment of malaria. The problem of resistance of *P. falciparum* to chloroquine is most serious in Western Kenya and along the Coast. Cases of multiple-drug resistance (i.e., resistance to drugs other than chloroquine) are also increasing across the continent.

It is important to note that infection of humans by malaria parasites need not lead to malarial illnesses. On the contrary, the infection may be a source of immunity against malaria. "Malarial morbidity declines at high levels of transmission" (Snow *et al.*, 1997). However, once malaria infection has developed into a disease, its treatment is the key control option, as prevention of healthy people from infection is merely a containment measure. Thus, information on costs, use and efficacy of malaria drugs is key in the success of malaria control efforts.

2.3.2 Institutions and malaria transmission

Institutions are formal rules (laws and regulations) and informal restrictions on behavior (traditions, customs shared values and beliefs) which structure interactions and relations among people (North, 1990). Regarding informal institutions, cultural norms as to types of housing, hours for social interaction and recreation, religious practices, and sex and age group occupations can play a major role in the transmission of malaria, and in determining which population subgroups suffer most from malaria. For example, fishermen who go out at night when certain types of mosquitoes are active are likely to contract malaria more often than other subgroups. Communal sleeping habits may also be a source of malaria.

Formal institutions such as public health regulations that allow the operation of certain businesses in residential areas without proper safeguards may also create an environment that is conducive to malaria transmission. For example, slaughter houses that are not properly kept can be breeding sites for mosquitoes. Uncollected garbage from licensed businesses in urban residential areas can serve the same purpose as well as national laws that establish irrigation schemes that create large reservoirs of malaria vectors. Information on the role played by informal and formal institutions in the transmission of malaria would be most valuable in its control.

2.4 A Historical Digression on Malaria Control

It is widely speculated that Africa is the origin of malaria, an Italian word meaning the disease of marshes or swamps (Bruce-Chwatt, 1986). Unfortunately, the malaria situation in Africa has generally remained static for decades. Despite successful control efforts in other world regions, there have been limited successes in only a few parts of Africa. Indeed, the earliest attempts in the world to control malaria were in Sierra Leone, West Africa in 1899 (Bruce-Chwatt, 1986).

A large-scale control of malaria (with the aim of eventual eradication) was launched by the World Health Organization (WHO) in 1955. In 1957, the World Health Assembly of WHO established and supported a world-wide malaria eradication program which lasted until 1969. At the end of the program the goal was revised from eradication to control because the eradication goal had proved infeasible. However, even though the program did not achieve its intended goal of global eradication of malaria, its direct and indirect effects are credited with the elimination of malaria from Southern United States, Europe, some parts of Middle East, North Africa and certain areas in South America. It is worth noting that substantial reductions in malaria prevalence had been achieved in the world prior to WHO's eradication and control programs, thanks to economic development (Hammer, 1993).

In 1978, the 31st World Health Assembly of WHO reoriented the malaria control program following the recommendations of the International Conference of Primary Health Care, held at Alma Ata in the same year. While community participation was given a prominent role in malaria control programs of countries, there was no global support unlike in the 1950s and 1960s. More recently, however, the UNDP/World Bank/WHO Special Program for Research and Training in Tropical Diseases (TDR) established in 1975, has devoted attention to the development of malaria vaccine and more effective anti-malarial drugs.

To date, no centralized, global program of malaria control exists. Much of the control work in tropical developing countries is being carried out indirectly by TDR, through its program of research and training on tropical diseases, one of which is malaria. Further, even though malarious countries in Africa and elsewhere have their own malaria control programs, these generally lack national outlook or are poorly organized. Recently, loose coalitions of international organizations have generated national level interests in malaria control in Africa because of a rising incidence in malaria in the region. Prominent among these is MIM (Multilateral Initiative on Malaria), an alliance of organizations and individuals concerned with malaria, whose aim is to maximize the impact of scientific research against malaria in Africa. The other partnership coalition is the Roll Back Malaria, a global initiative of the WHO and other development agencies; it sponsors collaborative action to help countries achieve their own goals against malaria.

This brief historical background should be helpful in constructively thinking about and designing malaria control programs in Africa. As this short background on global control efforts shows, an Africa-wide program of malaria control would not be in line with the current thinking about control strategies. Experience with large-scale malaria control programs also suggests that such a continent-level program would have little chance of success.

The most promising entry point, with regard to the control effort, is with existing national level malaria control programs. Such programs can be initiated where they do not exist; they can also be reoriented, reorganized and revitalized where they exist. Research on the situation (coverage, financing, strategies) of existing national malaria control programs would generate valuable information for reforming these programs and improving their performance.

2.5 Poverty-malaria Nexus

We start by considering the relationships between malaria and poverty at the macro level and then examine common underlying causes of the two phenomena. The discussion of the relationships is motivated by the following questions. What is the effect of poverty reduction on malaria? What is the effect of malaria control on poverty? These questions do not admit simple answers. To the extent that income poverty can be viewed merely as the absence of wealth, the two questions are concerned with the effect of growth on malaria and vice-versa.

2.5.1 The effect of poverty alleviation on malaria

Given the mechanics for generating growth, i.e., for poverty alleviation and the epidemiology of malaria, poverty reduction and malaria may be positively correlated at the early stages of economic development (Mwabu, 1991). That is, an increase in poverty reduction (e.g., a fall in the headcount ratio) may be accompanied by an increase in malaria prevalence. However, when poverty reduction reaches a certain critical level, malaria prevalence begins to decline with poverty reduction. This U-shaped relationship between poverty alleviation and malaria, is in contradiction with the simple hypothesis that poverty is the cause of malaria. The apparent contradiction arises from the fact that malaria can be on the increase even as poverty is reduced.

It is important to stress that the U-shaped relationship arises from the interaction of particular mechanics for poverty reduction with conditions conducive to malaria transmission. This possibly counterintuitive point is best illustrated with an example. The bulk of poverty in Africa is concentrated in rural, agricultural areas. In a semi-arid rural area, some of the mechanics for poverty reduction (for increasing agricultural incomes) include the introduction of irrigation schemes and construction of feeder roads to facilitate the marketing of farm produce.

Other things being equal, both of these transformations of an agricultural economy (via irrigated farming and public feeder roads) would lead to higher incomes and to lower poverty. However, the same transformations would create favorable conditions for malaria transmission and epidemics. The irrigation scheme, for example, would provide ideal mosquito breeding sites, while public feeder roads would facilitate quick transmission of malaria parasites from one area to another via movement of people and vectors.

During this early stage of development, people's response to increased malaria pathogens may be ineffective or lacking altogether. In that event, structural changes that make for higher incomes would reduce poverty but increase malaria incidence. However, as the decline in poverty rate reaches some threshold level, malaria infections and maladies may also decline due to effective control measures eventually developed by communities, reinforced by immunity acquired through exposure to malaria. It should be noted that poverty reduction strategies that do not affect malaria vector or malaria transmission would have a different outcome.

The foregoing discussion suggests that the malaria-poverty relationship is not a simple one, and may be uncovered only with certain kinds of data and modeling.

2.5.2 The effect of malaria control on poverty

It is now a short step to show that the poverty-malaria relationship is also not a linear one. Much of the recent literature on malaria and economic growth stresses the growth dividend of malaria control, i.e., increased poverty reduction due to malaria control. There may be no such dividend from malaria control or eradication. This does not imply that malaria control is not beneficial. The consumption benefits would be large, because the pain and suffering from malaria would be averted. However, production effects could be zero or negative. Avoidance of malaria by closing an irrigation scheme illustrates both cases of zero and negative effects. If benefits from loss of labor time due to malaria are equal to land productivity associated with an irrigation scheme, closure of the scheme would have no effect on total production. If, however, land productivity is greater than the opportunity cost of the time lost to malaria, closure of the scheme would reduce total income. Further, the counterfactual case where irrigation scheme is not built because of unbearable risks of malaria need not be associated with higher incomes. In that case, people would be free from malaria and yet might be poor. More generally, if the methods of malaria control are not cost-effective or efficient, the net production effects of the control may be negative or zero.

2.6 Proximate Determinants of Malaria and Poverty

Our working hypothesis is that poverty and malaria have a common set of underlying causes. Foremost among these are factors that precondition social and policy environment. These factors include climate, physical reality, biological endowments of individuals, cultural heritage (preferences, beliefs, and attitudes), and external shocks such as changes in foreign assistance, and in prices of key exports and pharmaceuticals.

The preconditioning factors directly determine a country's rate of growth and the quality of its health infrastructure, and hence its ability to institute effective malaria control and poverty alleviation programs. The preconditioning factors may affect behavior of the population in ways that are conducive to malaria transmission. For instance, given the structure of export prices, or the existing land policy, households might engage in cultivation practices that place them at high risks of malaria. Prevailing geographic conditions may also motivate households to behave in ways that are similarly risky.

2.7 Economic and Epidemiological Considerations in Malaria Control

2.7.1 Integrating economics with epidemiology

The economic approach to malaria control needs to take into account the epidemiological dimension of the disease as well. In designing disease control measures, knowledge about geographic and social profiles of a disease is as important as information about cost-effectiveness of control measures. "The potential for integrating economic and epidemiological reasoning in the formulation of policy for malaria control is great and largely untapped" (Hammer 1993:2). Epidemiological analysis of the disease helps define the bounds of the possible in its control, whereas economic analysis helps understand how people would respond to control measures. Also, choice of cost-effective and efficient measures of control are greatly facilitated by economic analysis. Needless to say, sociological and other knowledge bases are critical too in the design and choice of control instruments. These other disciplines have not been emphasized here because of limitations of space and expertise. We now consider the economic rationale for public action against malaria.

2.7.2 Economic rationale for public interventions against malaria

The rate of malaria transmission depends on the reservoir of malaria parasites in the population. The greater the reservoir, the higher is the probability of an individual in the population being infected and eventually contracting malaria. In seeking treatment, therefore, the individual reduces the level of the reservoir and hence the probability of infecting another person. However, an individual with a malarial illness cares only about the personal benefits to be derived from curing his own condition. In curing his condition, the individual does not consider the benefits s/he confers to others by reducing their probability of contracting malaria. Because of large positive social externalities associated with successful treatment or prevention of malaria, individuals under-invest in anti-malarial activities. To avoid such a situation, anti-malarial activities are best undertaken by public authorities.

Malaria can also be viewed as a public bad in another way. To the extent that malaria reduces productivity and taxable income, it erodes the general tax revenue of the government. Thus, it weakens the ability of the government to provide for social services. Public interventions to control and prevent malaria are therefore warranted on social considerations. Malaria as a public bad has no national boundaries because of the nature of malaria transmission. Eradication of malaria in one region or country would be short-lived if malaria is prevalent in contiguous regions or countries. Thus, malaria control programs should be organized collaboratively by regional as well as national authorities. The externalities associated with malaria should always be considered in the design of malaria control programs. We examine below applications of principles of malaria control from the perspectives of epidemiology and economics. We start with a brief examination of the epidemiological principles of malaria control.

2.7.3 Principles of malaria control

The control of malaria may be at the individual level (e.g., protection of one person) or at the community level (e.g., protection of the whole community). Measures for malaria control may be divided into five groups (Russell 1952; as cited in Bruce-Chwatt 1986) as follows:

(a) measures designed to prevent mosquitoes from feeding on people;
(b) measures designed to prevent or reduce the breeding of mosquitoes by eliminating the collections of water or by altering the environment;
(c) measures designed to destroy the larvae of mosquitoes;
(d) measures designed to destroy adult mosquitoes; and
(e) measures designed to eliminate the malaria parasites in the human host.

Table 2.1 summarizes the types of malaria control measures and their associated effects on malaria vectors and vector habitats.

The above principles of control are sound in theory but their effective implementation, especially in Africa, has proved difficult. To facilitate economic assessment of various measures, we provide a brief description of the elements of some of the measures.

2.7.4 Protection against mosquito bites

Protective devices and measures against mosquito bites include bed nets, protective clothing, repellents, screening of windows or dwellings, and selection of suitable site for new housing. Bed nets are some of the most important measures for personal protection against mosquito bites. Insecticide sprayed on nets has recently been shown to be quite effective in killing mosquitoes (Goodman and Mills, 1999). Boots, thick socks or trousers can be used as protection against mosquito bites in the evening or during night duty.

Repellents are substances applied to the skin, clothing or bed nets to repel mosquitoes and prevent them from biting. There are many varieties of these substances, varying by effectiveness and duration of protection. Screening of dwellings or of windows is an effective protection against

Table 2.1 Principles of comprehensive malaria control

Type of control	Effect
*Individual protection**	
Mosquito repellents	Reduction of man-mosquito contact
Bed nets	
House screening	
House siting	
Pyrethrum house spraying	
Anti-mosquito fumigants	
*Vector control**	
Environment modification and manipulation	Reduction of vector breeding habitats
Chemical and biological larvicides	Reduction of vector densities
Insecticide space spraying	Reduction of longevity of vector population
Residue insecticide spraying	
*Antiplasmodial measures***	
Treatment of acute cases of malaria	Elimination of malaria parasites and prevention of transmission
Prophylaxis and suppression of malaria infection	
Radical treatment of relapses	
Vaccination against malaria	

* Factors reducing the vectorial capacity.
** Factors reducing the parasite reservoir.

Source: Bruce-Chwatt (1986, p. 265).

mosquitoes. More recently, impregnated mosquito curtains (Rubardt *et al.*, 1999) have been shown to have high perceived efficacy in malaria control in Malawi.

Prudent selection of sites for new housing can avoid subsequent costs of treatments for malaria. The house should be placed upwind from the nearest water source. It should also be at least a mile from such a source to reduce mosquito breeding sites in the vicinity of a house.

In some areas or countries, households might be using some of the above methods of personal protection on their own or as a result of incentives from the government. However, in some communities, proven devices of protection such as impregnated bed nets may never have been tried. A study of people's preferences over the various methods of protection would help identify why effective methods are not being used in certain contexts. A study on the role of costs in the adoption of control methods would be valuable to policy makers in ministries of health.

2.7.5 Mosquito control and eradication

Methods of mosquito control include alteration of mosquito breeding sites (species sanitation); destruction of adult mosquitoes with insecticides; anti-larval measures, and use of biological agents such as fish that feed on mosquitoes. Changing mosquito breeding habitats through engineering measures may be very difficult and expensive to accomplish in some areas. Mosquito control through residue spraying can be effective but has very undesirable environmental consequences. The disease vectors may also develop resistance against commonly used insecticides. However, the basic goal of insecticide spraying is not to kill all Anopheles mosquitoes at once but to prevent a large proportion of them from surviving beyond a certain period.

Biological methods of mosquito may be applied to mosquito control. They involve the introduction into the environment predators of the insect vectors of malaria. Effective application of these methods though requires good knowledge of the bionomics of the vector species and of the local ecological conditions.

2.7.6 Elimination of malaria parasites from human host and prevention of malaria infection

Chemotherapy and chemoprophylaxis are the methods used to remove malaria parasites from the human host or to prevent malaria parasites injected into a human body from developing into a disease. Chemotherapy refers to use of drugs to cure malaria maladies, while chemoprophylaxis is the use of drugs for protection against malaria attack. Some drugs serve curative and protective purposes. For example, chloroquine can be used both as a chemotherapeutic (curative) and as a prophylactic (protective) drug. A protective drug is taken before a malaria infection, while a curative one is taken after the infection.

An analysis of markets for malaria chemotherapy and chemoprophylaxis would provide important information for formulation of anti-malaria policy.

Throughout Sub-Saharan Africa, there are numerous market outlets for malaria drugs of various types (see Musonda and Mangani, this volume).

2.7.7 Control and eradication of malaria

In closing this section, it is important to point out differences between malaria control and malaria eradication. The distinction is important because it should help policymakers in each country to decide whether given their resource and technological constraints, they want to go for malaria control or eradication. The presentation here is based on Bruce-Chwatt (1986).

The objective of malaria eradication is to stop transmission and eliminate the human reservoir of infection altogether, while control is intended to reduce malaria incidence until the disease is no longer a major public health problem. Eradication is undertaken within a limited time period; in contrast control has an indefinite time duration. Malaria eradication is pursued in all areas where the disease occurs, while control is undertaken only where transmission is intense. In the case of eradication, recurrent costs are minimal after completion of the campaign, since national malaria activity is limited to malaria surveillance only. Capital costs for eradication, however, can be large and unaffordable by many countries. In the control case, capital costs are not as large, but cumulative recurrent expense is large because it is incurred practically over an indefinite period.

It is confusing to view malaria control and eradication as two distinct goals because malaria control is the intermediate outcome of the eradication goal. When the social goal is malaria eradication, resources are spent on eradication activities until malaria is eliminated altogether from the population. The assumption in this case is that the net marginal social benefit from eradication of the last malaria parasite is positive or zero. If, however, the net marginal social benefit is negative (i.e., the cost of eliminating the last parasite is greater than the associated benefit), eradication effort stops at the control stage. It is for each country to decide, based on net marginal social benefit calculation, whether its approach to malaria menace should be an eradication or a control strategy. In any case, the eradication decision should be made after the intermediate goal of control has been achieved. It is pointless for a country to set for itself an eradication goal when it does not have the means to achieve the control goal. Regional groupings such as East Africa or Southern Africa should make malaria control and eradication decisions using similar reasoning as at national levels.

2.7.8 Malaria vaccine and malaria control & eradication

The availability of malaria vaccine would not substantially alter the malaria control scenario described above. Whether or not application of the vaccine would eradicate malaria would depend on the extent of application. If a sufficiently large proportion of the population were to be effectively immunized against malaria, malaria would be eradicated. However, the net marginal social benefit of the extra immunization coverage (i.e., the coverage that would ensure eradication) may be negative. In that case, the vaccine would be used to control rather than to eradicate malaria. The interesting aspect of control or eradication here is that attention would be turned away from malaria vectors. With the vaccine, Anopheles mosquito bites would only be a nuisance to people but would transmit no disease.

2.8 Malaria Burden in Children

It has already been noted that around one million children in Africa die every year from malaria and more than 300 million people suffer from mosquito bites each year. Around ten per cent of the total disease burden in Africa (measured in disability adjusted life years lost) is due to malaria (Goodman and Mills, 1999). Further, over eighty eight per cent of the world malaria burden falls on Africans.

This section focuses on malaria burden in children in Africa, the population group most affected by malaria. In addition to malaria incidence being highest among children, malaria mortality is also highest among children. Highlighting these issues is particularly important for poverty reduction. Malaria burden is positively correlated with poverty: malaria index risk is highest in low-income countries in the tropics, with Africa accounting for a preponderance of these countries.

Snow *et al.*, (1999) have used a combination of methods to estimate malaria mortality and morbidity rates for Africa. The authors calculated the risk of malaria transmission in different parts of Africa on a scale of zero to one on the basis of recorded climatic data and prior knowledge of the effects of different climatic variables on mosquito survival and parasite development. A malaria suitability climate of zero indicates that the region is not conducive to the development of malaria and hence malaria risk in the area is zero. A climatic index of one shows that the region is ideal for malaria parasites and hence the population in the region is exposed to high risks of malaria. As shown in table 2.2, malaria risks for children differ even for the same climatic index depending on region, which is an indication of high regional specificity of malaria risks.

Among areas located within climate suitable for malaria, a suitability index of greater than zero but less than 0.5 for Southern Africa and less than 0.2 for the rest of Sub-Saharan Africa, indicates the overall risks of disease and death that are unusually large. In malaria endemic areas and those with high malaria transmission, nearly 100 million children under the age of five face high risks of malaria morbidity and mortality. The table shows that children under the age of five years bear a disproportionately high burden of malaria morbidity, a point emphasized further in table 2.3. For example, the risk of celebral malaria is higher among the 0–4 year olds than among children in age bracket 5–9 years. For the under-fives, around 0.1815 per cent of children in the general population are admitted to the hospital compared to 0.0345 per cent for older age group. In other words, the probability that a zero to four year old will be admitted to a hospital with celebral malaria (0.182%) is about six times higher than the probability of a five to nine year old (0.035%) being admitted with the same condition. Assuming that all children have an equal chance of being taken to the hospital for malaria treatment, these risk probabilities show that the under-fives face a higher risk of malaria than older children. However, the five to nine year-olds with severe malaria anaemia have higher risks of contracting HIV from blood transfusions than the under-fives (Table 2.3).

As can be seen from table 2.3, the availability of health care services (especially proximity to a hospital) cuts down risks of celebral malaria among all children, particularly the under-fives. This is perhaps a reflection of a low vectorial capacity in those population groups that are within easy access to malaria treatments at a hospital. The finding underscores the importance of having broadly available basic health services for the success of malaria control programs. The availability of basic health services is important because malaria occurs in conjunction with other diseases such as diarrhea, AIDS, tuberculosis and pneumonia. These diseases need to be treated or

Table 2.2 Population and mortality estimates for the interpolated distribution of people according to classifications of transmission risk (interquartile range in parentheses)

Population Group	African population exposed to different malaria risks (excluding Southern and Northern Africa)			Southern African population	
	0 climate suitability: No malaria risk	>0 and < 0.2 climate suitability: Epidemic malaria risk	>0.2 climate suitability: Stable transmission	<0.5 climate suitability: No malaria risk area	>0.5 climate suitability: Malaria risk area
Population aged 0-4 years	4,609,524	9,850,391	81,429,978	5,504,839	3,025,494
Median mortality rate per 1000 population	–	na	9.4 (7.1, 12.4)	–	0.11 (0.02, 0.20)
Estimated numbers of deaths in 1995	0	na	765,442	0	333
Same as above	–	–	(57,8153–1,009,732)	(61-605)	–
Population aged 5-9 years	3,770,381	8,174,807	67,032,624	4,893,730	2,6,02,153
Median mortality rate per 1000 population	–	na	2.17 (1.64, 2.86)	–	0.1 (0.02. 0.20)
Estimated numbers of deaths in 1995	0	na	145,461	0	286
Same	–	–	(109,934–191,713)	–	(52-520)
Population aged 10-14 years	3,097,257	6,906,370	56,360,964	453,5489	2,359,704
Median mortality rate per 1000 population	–	na	0.80 (0.61, 1.06)	–	0.11 (0.02. 0.20)

Continued

Table 2.2 *(continued)*

Population Group	African population exposed to different malaria risks (excluding Southern and Northern Africa)			Southern African population	
	0 climate suitability: No malaria risk	**>0 and < 0.2 climate suitability: Epidemic malaria risk**	**>0.2 climate suitability Stable transmission**	**<0.5 climate suitability: No malaria risk area**	**>0.5 climate suitability Malaria risk area**
Estimated numbers of deaths in 1995	0	na	45089	–	260
Same	–	–	(34,380–59,743)	–	(47–472)
Population aged > 15 years	13,329,952	29,639,097	242,110,974	2,417,9130	1,142,2561
Median mortality rate per 1000 population	–	na	0.13 (0.09, 0.17)	–	0.11 (0.02, 0.20)
Estimated numbers of deaths in 1995	0	na	31,474	0	1256
Same	–	–	(21,790–41,159)	–	(228–2285)
Total population in 1995	24,807,114	54,570,668	446,934,540	39,113,188	19,409,912
Total deaths in 1995 [non-epidemic year]	0	na	987466	0	2135
Same	–	–	(744,257–1,302,347)	–	–

Source: Snow et al., (1999).

prevented even as malaria is controlled. Thus, strengthening primary health care should be a key element of a malaria control program.

The epidemiological definitions of unstable or epidemic malaria do not reflect the public health significance of the disease for these regions of Africa. Nevertheless, it is agreed that the risks of disease and death from malaria

Table 2.3 Sequelae risks and events following admission to hospital among children living in stable endemic areas of Africa (interquartile range in parentheses)

Outcome	Age group in years	
	0–4	**0–9**
Risk of celebral malaria admission from communities within 15km of a hospital (*per 1000 population per annum*).	1.815 (0.26, 2.60)	0.345 (0.13,0.61)
Risk of surviving hospitalization with celebral malaria.	1.472 (0.211, 2.11)	0.280 (0.11,0.495)
Risk of surviving hospitalization with celebral malaria, allowing for the proportion of population within 15 km of hospital.	0.528 (0.076, 0.756)	0.101 (0.040,0.178)
Neurological sequelae risk of residual effects after six months (*per 1000 children per annum*).	0.030 (0.004, 0.042)	0.006 (0.002,0.010)
Number of neurological sequelae events (figures in brackets are the range).	2443 [356–3420]	402 [134–670]
Risk of severe malaria anaemia admission from communities within 15 km of a hospital (*per 1000 population per annum*).	7.61 (3.99, 11.61)	0.47 (0.11, 0.72)
Risk of surviving hospitalization with severe malaria anaemia and receiving blood transfusion (*per 1000 population p.a.*).	4.81 (2.52,7.34)	0.29 (0.007, 0.46)
Risk of surviving hospitalization with transfused severe malaria anaemia, allowing for proportion of population within 15 km of a hospital (*per 1000 population per annum*).	1.73 (0.905, 2.640	0.10 (0.003,0.165)
Risk of survivors with severe malaria anaemia who had a blood transfusion, who acquire HIV when background risks apply to those in Kinshasa in late 1980s (*per 1000 pop p.a.*).	0.225 (0.118,0.343)	0.013 (0.0004,0.022)
Number of HIV events arising from blood transfusions of severe malaria anaemia (figures in brackets are the range).	18.322 [9609–27930]	871.00 [29–1475]

Source: Snow et al., (1999).

are dependent upon a wide range of factors including protective genetic constitution of individuals, acquired immunity; access to and use of curative services; drug resistance of parasites; and protective behaviors of communities against infection. These factors vary across the African continent, resulting in significant differences in disease outcomes between areas. The most significant factor is the interplay between the age of acquired functional immunity under stable transmission conditions, and risks of mortality.

The challenge for most African households is that of proper timing in the effective application of barrier methods such as the intensive use of impregnated bed nets during the rainy season. The knowledge of epidemiological characteristics of the mosquito in a given region is also important in people's self-protection against malaria. The immunological responsiveness of a population group by age and area is another determinant of the outcome of malaria infection. In holoendemic areas, malaria contributes significantly to child mortality and can cause acute disease in pregnant women, but does not have large effects on the fitness of other mature adults due to their partial immunity acquired through constant re-infection.

When it comes to health and survival risks, nothing is of greater concern in many poor African countries as the lack of medical services and insufficient provisions for malaria treatments. The problem here is not merely the lack of effective medical remedies. Sen (1999) notes that the failure to treat effectively applies to perfectly treatable diseases such as cholera and common malaria, as well as more challenging ailments such as AIDS, and drug-resistant malaria and tuberculosis. Sen suggests that public interventions that could make a difference against deprivations that keep people ill and poor, be implemented and sustained.

2.9 Economic Studies on Malaria in Africa

Why study malaria from an economic perspective? Malaria as a societal problem has several dimensions that economic analysis can help illuminate. The potential and actual economic burdens of malaria, due to loss in fiscal revenue and labor productivity have already been noted. Assessment of these burdens, including how they can be alleviated, is an important step in the design of programs for improving standards of living in Africa. It has also been noted that a large proportion of the African population suffers from malaria annually. The resources spent on treating malaria can be put to other uses if malaria were to be eliminated or controlled to tolerable levels.

Economic analysis can assist in estimating the magnitude of benefits that can be derived from successful control efforts and thus give impetus to such efforts. Resources for combating malaria are severely limited in Africa. It is, therefore, critical to find cost-effective methods of malaria control or eradication. Economic research, especially in collaborative form, can greatly contribute to this endeavor. Scarcity of health resources in Africa is probably the main reason for many studies on cost-effectiveness of malaria control programs undertaken in the region since the 1960s.

Cost-effectiveness studies attempt to provide answers to the following sorts of questions. Which malaria control strategies are most effective and what are their costs? What alternatives exist to improve malaria treatments, and how much does each cost? What are the returns to investments in malaria control, and how do the returns compare with those from competing investments? These questions can be asked at the household level, at the level of the community, or at the national level. They are important questions to answer whenever scarce resources are being spent, especially on a large scale.

Goodman and Mills (1999) identified and evaluated fourteen studies on cost-effectiveness of malaria control strategies in Africa dating from the early 1970s. The majority of the studies (11) provided information on cost-effectiveness of insecticide treated bed nets, residual spraying, chemoprophylaxis for children, and intermittent treatment for pregnant women. Two studies estimated cost-effectiveness of a hypothetical vaccine. However, no cost-effectiveness analysis was reported for untreated bed nets; other methods of personal protection (such as coils and sprays); environmental management; or the control of epidemics. Such studies should be undertaken and their cost-effectiveness ratios compared with ratios from treated bed nets for example. Table 2.4 provides a list of interventions whose cost-effectiveness studies in Africa are evaluated.

The third and fourth columns of table 2.4 show costs of various interventions per unit of outcome (child death averted or discounted year of life gained).

Since these are costs per unit of outcome, they can also be read as cost-effectiveness ratios. Although other outcome measures such as "number of malaria free days per year" or "number of school absences averted" can be used, these might have the disadvantage of lacking international comparability. Thus, internationally comparable outcome measures such as the number of disability adjusted years, child averted deaths or discounted life years gained should be used whenever possible.

According to table 2.4, costs of interventions vary considerably from one country to another and also for the same country. In two trials that involved the provision of nets and two treatments per year in Ghana and Kenya, the Ghana trial was more cost-effective than the Kenyan trial. In Kenya, the cost per child death averted was approximately US$ 2958 while in Ghana, the cost was US$ 2112.

Effectiveness may also vary due to differences in epidemiological conditions, demographic factors, immunity levels and drug resistance (Goodman and Mills, 1999). For example, disparities in schooling levels and cultural factors, such as beliefs about the cause of malaria and how best to treat the disease, can affect compliance with the intervention and hence its effectiveness. Changes of these cultural factors over time can substantially alter the cost-effectiveness ratios of interventions, with methods that were originally cost-effective becoming ineffective and vice-versa. Thus, dynamic rather than static cost-effectiveness ratios would provide better guides for policy.

Reviewing cost-effectiveness studies on Africa, Goodman and Mills (1999) conclude that despite variations in results obtained, highly cost effective interventions for malaria control exist in Africa. In a highly informative summary of results from cost-effectiveness research in low income Africa (Goodman 1999) lists the cost per disability-adjusted-life year at US$1995 as follows:

- $4–10 for insecticide treatment of existing mosquito nets;
- $19–85 for provision of mosquito nets and insecticide treatment;
- $16–29 for residual house spraying with one round a year, and $32–58 with two rounds;
- $3–12 for chemoprophylaxis for children under five years (assuming an existing system for intervention delivery);

Table 2.4 Cost-effectiveness results for interventions against malaria using comparable outcome measures (figures in parentheses are ranges in cost estimates)

Type of Intervention	Country & year	Cost of the Outcome Achieved by the Intervention (Constant 1995 US Dollars)	
		Cost per Child Death Averted ($)	Cost per Discounted Year Life Gained ($)
Insecticide treatment of bed nets	The Gambia (1989–90)	219 (167–243)	9(9–14)
Insecticide treatment of bed nets and chemoprophylaxis	The Gambia (1989–90)	300 (246–333)	13(13–20)
Insecticide treatment of bed nets	The Gambia (1991–92)	494 (326–805)	21(14–35)
Provision and insecticide treatment of bed nets	Ghana (1993–95)	2112 (992–2289)	77(37–84)
Provision and insecticide treatment of bed nets	Kenya (1993–94)	2958 (2838–3120)	na
Provision and insecticide treatment of bed nets	Africa :(1996); using Gambia cost data	na	10–118
Insecticide treatment of bed nets	The Gambia (1990)	829 (447–2117)	na
Hypothetical Vaccine	The Gambia (1990)	294 (163–737)	na
Hypothetical Vaccine	Africa (1996)	na	0.36–41 (High transmission)
Hypothetical Vaccine	Africa	na	5–621 (Low transmission)
Chemoprophylaxis for children	The Gambia (1988)	167	na

Continued

Table 2.4 *(continued)*

Type of Intervention	Country & year	Cost of the Outcome Achieved by the Intervention (Constant 1995 US Dollars)	
		Cost per Child Death Averted ($)	Cost per Discounted Year Life Gained ($)
Antenatal treatment and chemoprophylaxis:2 Sulfadoxine-Pyrimethamine (SP) treatments	Malawi (1992)	81(79–352)	na
1 SP treatment, weekly chloroquine chemoprophylaxis (CQ)	Malawi (1992)	522 (212–812)	na
1 CQ treatment, weekly CQ prophylaxis	Malawi (1992)	950 (317–951)	na
Drug treatment for children: CQ (No resistance scenario)	Africa (1991)	1.47 (0.21–3.36)	na
CQ (Low resistance scenario)	Africa (1991)	1.49 (0.22–3.36)	na
CQ (High resistance scenario)	Africa (1991)	2.56 (0.31–4.34)	na
Amodiaquine, AQ (No and low resistance scenarios)	Africa (1991)	2.35 (0.34–5.40)	na
AQ (High resistance scenario)	Africa (1991)	2.89 (0.40–5.67)	na
SP (All resistance scenarios)	Africa (1991)	1.70 (0.25–3.92)	na

Source: Goodman and Mills (1999), Table 2, pp. 308–9.

- $14–93 for weekly chloroquine chemoprophylaxis for primigravidae pregnant women, and $4–29 for intermittent treatment with sulfadoxine-pyrimethamine;
- $2–8 for improving compliance with treatment through training providers, educating patients and care-takers, and prepackaging of chloroquine; and
- $0.7–3 for improving the availability of second and third line of drugs for treatment failures.

If US$150 is taken as an acceptable or the "standard" cost-effectiveness ratio (Goodman, 1999), it is clear that the above interventions are highly cost-effective. Even so, there is need to confirm these results in different African settings. It should also be noted that the cost-effectiveness results tend to inform mainly the supply-side interventions. In particular, though the results help identify the appropriate intervention packages to be delivered to the population, the demand side of malaria control effort, that is, how the population responds to interventions has not received as much attention.

2.10 Conclusion

The chapter has provided a framework for understanding the interrelationships between malaria and poverty in Africa. It has described the state of malaria in Africa, including its transmission mechanisms and control methods. In addition, the chapter has provided a historical account of global malaria control and eradication efforts, which serve as a backdrop to current country-specific control programs.

Several gaps in the information required to design and implement malaria control programs in African countries have been identified. Information on demand for malaria control services and products is particularly lacking. Also lacking is knowledge of effects of malaria on labor productivity in agricultural and industrial settings, as well as on settlement and farming patterns. Although cost-effectiveness information is available, it is restricted to impregnated bed nets. There is need therefore to compute cost-effectiveness ratios for other methods of control. The methodology for undertaking cost-effectiveness analysis with results that can be compared internationally is not well established or well known.

We have established that provision of basic health services is an important factor in the control of malaria. The synergy between national primary health care programs and the national malaria control programs needs to be investigated. Also lacking is information about national delivery systems for malaria drugs, as well as optimal procurement procedures for these drugs. Models of economic and social effects of malaria are grossly lacking. In particular, the connection between malaria and poverty is not well understood. It has been established in the African context and elsewhere that education is a key determinant of poverty status of households (Fosu, Mwabu, Thorbeceke, 2003). Since malaria and poverty appear to be closely linked, there is need to examine the effect of education on malaria more closely.

One place to start in the control of malaria in Africa would be an understanding of the existing national malaria control programs. Information on management, financing, and performance of these programs would be useful in implementing reforms to improve the programs or in designing new ones.

In-depth household level economic studies of malaria in Africa are lacking. Recently, many countries in Africa have undertaken living standard measurement type surveys, which provide information about malaria infections and the treatment options pursued by households. These surveys can be used to examine demand patterns for malaria treatment. Intrahousehold distribution of malaria treatments can be examined using the same surveys. Since malaria accounts for a large disease burden in Africa, it is important to determine whether there is bias in intrahousehold distribution of malaria drugs, treatments, and preventive devices such as the bed nets and mosquito coils. Such information would be useful in deciding whether or not to target particular household members for malaria treatment or prevention.

Existing household survey data can be used to understand the distribution of malaria in a given country, including the characteristics of people most afflicted by the disease. Where such surveys do not exist, rapid household and facility surveys can be undertaken to provide information about strategies currently being used to deal with malaria. Ideally, the surveys should be designed to collect household and community level information that is likely to be of relevance to malaria control. For example, at the household level, information can be collected about malaria episodes, perceived causes of the disease, and treatment strategies implemented by households, including, the social and economic effects of malaria.

At the community level, information can be obtained about characteristics of treatment facilities (quality of services, availability of staff and drugs), and distances to sources of water, schools and other public amenities. If the major problem of poverty is to be addressed successfully in Africa, control and eventual eradication of malaria are required. The chapters by Mwabu (2007), Olagoke (2007), Kamgnia (2007), and Musonda and

Mangani (2007) in this volume offer country-specific accounts of malaria situations and control efforts in Africa.

References

African Medical and Research Foundation (AMREF) (1996), *Towards Self Sufficiency*. Nairobi: AMREF.

African Summit on Roll Back Malaria (2000), "Economic Analyzes Indicate that the Burden of Malaria is Great", African Summit on Roll Back Malaria, Abuja, Nigeria, Harvard University and London School of Hygiene and Tropical Medicine, April 2000.

Aikins, M.K., *et al.*, (1998), "The Gambian National Impregnated Bednet Program: Consequences and Net Cost-effectiveness". *Social Science and Medicine* 46 (2): 181–91.

Alonso, P.L., Lindsay, S.W., and Armstrong, J.R. (1991), "The Effect of Insecticide-treated Bed Nets on Mortality of Gambian Children". *Lancet* 337 (8756): 1499–502.

American Association for the Advancement of Science (1991), *Malaria and Development in Africa*. Washington, D.C.: American Association for the Advancement of Science.

Barlow, R., and Grobar, L.M. (1986), "Costs and Benefits of Controlling Parasitic Diseases". Washington, D.C.: Population, Health and Nutrition Department, The World Bank,

Binka, F.N., Mensah, O.A., and Mills, A. (1997), "The Cost-Effectiveness of Permethrin Impregnated Bednets in Preventing Child Mortality in Kassena-Nankana District of Northern Ghana". *Health Policy* 41: 220–9.

Brown, G. (1997), "Fighting Malaria". *British Medical Journal*, 314: 1707–1708.

Bruce-Chwatt, L.J. (1986), *Essential Malariology, Second Edition.* UK: William Heinemann Medical Books.

Cohn, E.J. (1973), "Assessing the Costs and Benefits of Antimalaria Programs: The Indian Experience". *American Journal of Public Health* 63: 1086–96.

Coleman, P.G., Goodman, C.A. and Mills, A.J. (1999), "Rebound Mortality and the Cost-Effectiveness of Malaria Control: Potential Impact of Increased Mortality in Late Childhood Following the Introduction of Insecticide Treated Nets". *Tropical Medicine and International Health* 4(3): 175–186.

Conly, G.N. (1975), "Thc Impact of Malaria on Economic Development: A Case Study". *Scientific Publication, 297.* Washington D.C: Pan American Health Organization.

D'Alessandro U., Olaleye, B.O., and McGuire, W. *et al.* (1995), "Mortality and Morbidity from Malaria in Gambian Children after Introduction of an Impregnated Bednet Program". *Lancet* 345 (8948): 479–83.

Evans, D.B., Azene, G., and Kirigia, J. (1997), "Should Government Subsidize the Use of Insecticide-Impregnated Mosquito Nets in Africa: Implications of a Cost-Effectiveness Analysis". *Health Policy and Planning* 12 (2): 107–14.

Filmer, D., and Pritchett, L. (1999), "The Effect of Household Wealth on Educational Attainment: Evidence from 35 Countries". *Population and Development Review* 25 (1): 85–120.

Foster, S.D. (1991), "Pricing, Distribution, and the Use of Anti-malarial Drugs". *Bulletin of the World Health Organization* 69 (3): 349–63.

Fosu, A.K., Mwabu, G. and Thorbecke, E. (2003), "Poverty in Africa", Unpublished Manuscript, AERC, Nairobi.

Gold, M.R *et al.*, (1996), *Cost-Effectiveness in Health and Medicine*. New York: Oxford University Press.

Goodman, C.A., and Mills, A.J. (1999), "The Evidence Base on the Cost-Effectiveness of Malaria Control Measures in Africa", *Health Policy and Planning* 14 (4): 301–312.

Goodman, C. (1999), "The Cost-Effectiveness of Malaria Control in Sub-Saharan Africa", *Briefing Notes, HEFP Briefing Note No. 7* (October). The London School of Hygiene and Tropical Medicine.

Goodman, C.A., Coleman, P.G. and Mills, A.J. (1999), "Cost-Effectiveness of Malaria Control in Sub-Saharan Africa". *Lancet* 354: 378–85.

Greenwood, B. (1999), "Malaria Mortality and Morbidity in Africa". *Bulletin of the World Health Organization* 77 (8): 617–618.

Hammer, J.S. (1992), "To Prescribe or Not to Prescribe: On the Regulation of Pharmaceuticals in Less Developed Countries". *Social Science and Medicine* 34 (9): 959–64.

Hammer, J.S. (1993), "The Economics of Malaria Control", *The World Bank Research Observer* 8 (1): 1–22.

Hanemann, W.M. (1991), "Willingness to Pay and Willingness to Accept: How much can they differ?". *American Economic Review* 81 (3): 635–47.

Jamison, D. *et al.*, (eds.) (1993), *Disease Control Priorities in Developing Countries*. New York: Oxford University Press.

Kamgnia, B. (2007), "The Demand for Malaria Control Products and Services: Evidence from Yaounde, Cameroon", this Volume.

KEMRI – Wellcome Trust (1999), *Malaria Situation Analysis for Kenya*. Nairobi: Kenya Medical Research Institute.

Mills, A. (1998), "Operational Research on the Economics of Insecticide-Treated Mosquito Nets: Lessons of Experience". *Annals of Tropical Medicine and Parasitology* 92 (4): 435–47.

Musonda, F.M. and Mangani, F. (2007), "The Distribution of Pharmaceutical Products and Malaria Control in Zambia", this Volume.

Mwabu, G. (1991), "Economic Development and Malaria Prevalence: An Empirical Analysis with Reference to Kenya" in *Malaria and Development in Africa*, Washington, D.C.: American Association for the Advancement of Science.

Najera, *et al.*, (1992), "Malaria: New Patterns and Perspectives", *Technical Paper 183*, Washington, D.C.: The World Bank.

Nevill, C.G. (1990), "Malaria in Sub-Saharan Africa", *Social Science and Medicine* 31 (6): 667–9.

Nevill, C.G., Some, E.S., and Munga'la, V.O., *et al.*, (1996), "Insecticide-Treated Bednets Reduce Mortality and Severe Morbidity from Malaria Among Children on the Kenyan Coast". *Tropical Medicine and International Health* 1 (2): 139–46.

North, D.C. (1990), *Institutions, Institutional Change and Economic Performance*. Cambridge: Cambridge University Press,

Omumbo, J., Ouma, J., Rapuoda, B., Craig, M.H., Le Sueur, D. and Snow, R.W. (1998), "Mapping Malaria Transmission Intensity Using Geographic Information Systems (GIS): An Example from Kenya". *Annals of Tropical Medicine & Parasitology* 92: pp. 7–21.

Olagoke, A.O. (2007), "The Economic Burden of Childhood Malaria in Nigeria", this Volume.

Onari, E. (1984), "The Problems of Plasmodium Drug Resistance in Africa South of the Sahara". *Bulletin of the World Health Organization* (Suppl) 62 (55).

Ongore, D. *et al.*, (1989), "A Study of Knowledge, Attitudes and Practices (KAP of a Rural Community on Malaria and the Mosquito Vector)". *East African Medical Journal*, Vol. 66: 79–90.

Rubardt, M., and Chikoko, A., *et al.*, (1999), "Implementing a Malaria Curtains Project in Malawi". *Health Policy and Planning* 14 (4): 313–321.

Sachs, J.D., and Gallup, L.J. (1999), "Malaria, Climate and Poverty, CAER II Discussion Paper No. 48, HIID", Harvard University.

Sen, A. (1999), "Health in Development". *Bulletin of the World Health Organization* 77 (8): 619–623.

Sharma, A.S. *et al.*, (1991), "The Kheda Malaria Project: The Case for Environmental Control". *Health Policy and Planning*, 6 (3): 262–270.

Sharma, V.P. and Mehrotra, K.N. "Malaria Resurgence in India: A Critical Study". *Social Science and Medicine* 22: 835–845.

Snow, R.W., Craig, M., Deichmann, U., and Marsh, K. (1999), "Estimating Mortality, Morbidity and Disability due to Malaria Among Africa's Non–Pregnant Population". *Bulletin of the World Health Organization* 77 (8): 624–640.

Snow, R.W., *et al.*, (1997), "Relation Between Severe Malaria Morbidity in Children and Level of *Plasmodium falciparum* Transmission in Africa". *Lancet* 349 (June 7): 1650–1654.

United Nations Children's Education Fund (UNICEF) (1991), *Malaria In Kenya – What Communities Can Do*. Nairobi: UNICEF Country Office.

Wiemer, C. (1987), "Optimal Disease Control through Combined use of Preventive and Curative Measures". *Journal of Development Economics* 25: 301–19.

World Health Organization (WHO) (1980), *Resistance of Vectors of Disease to Pesticides.* Tech. Rep. Serial No. 655, Geneva: World Health Organization.

World Bank (2000), *Can Africa Claim the 21st Century? Investing in People.* Washington, D.C.: World Bank.

Part II

Case Studies

Chapter 3

The Economic Burden of Malaria in Kenya

Germano Mwabu

3.0 Introduction

Malaria is a serious problem in Kenya and in other African countries. Approximately eighty to eighty five per cent of the cases of population morbidity and mortality in Sub-Saharan Africa are attributable to malaria (American Association for the Advancement of Science, 1991). However, since the mid-1990s, AIDS pandemic has increasingly contributed to population mortality and morbidity in the continent and its toll on African economies is mounting (Arndt and Lewis, 2000). Due to space limitation, economic effects of HIV/AIDS are not analyzed here, but to some extent, are indirectly considered in our measurement of economic burden of malaria relative to other diseases.

The malaria problem has at least three dimensions – the health, the social and the economic dimensions. The health problem is evidenced by high malaria-related mortality and morbidity in many African countries, Kenya included. Malaria deaths in Sub-Saharan Africa amount to some 0.5 to two million deaths per year, with children accounting for 0.75 to one million of these deaths (Snow *et al*., 1997; Okorosobo, 2000). The disease afflicts mainly pregnant women, young children, migratory populations and persons with little previous exposure to malaria attacks (Snow, *et al*., 1999).

Even though little is known about the social burden of malaria, there is evidence that social interaction of people and communities is hindered by risks of malaria (Gallup and Sachs, 2000). The economic dimension of the malaria problem, however, is closely linked to health and social dimensions. Social isolation of communities can inhibit transmission of new ideas and technologies and thus retard growth in incomes (Gallup and Sachs, 2000).

Malaria mortality and morbidity can also slow growth by reducing capacity and efficiency of the labor force in market and non-market environments.

Macroeconometric studies show a large economic burden of malaria in Africa and in specific countries in the region since the 1960s. In 1983 for example, economic growth in Kenya would have been 1.28 per cent higher if the country had been free from malaria (McCarthy, Wolf and Wu, 2000). A malaria free environment is conducive to economic growth for several reasons. First, it allows households to engage in efficient agricultural land-use practices rather than in labor-saving, low-productivity practices such as the planting of root crops whose yields are affected very little by malarial illnesses within households (Wang'ombe and Mwabu, 1993). Second, a malaria free environment encourages spatial labor mobility, an aspect that is conduce to diffusion of new technologies in society. A third and related point is that a malaria free country would attract investments in tourist industries (which are highly labor intensive) and thus help reduce unemployment. Fourth, healthy workers (or workers with less debilitating illnesses) are, other things being equal, more productive and more effective in acquiring work skills. Finally, in a malaria free environment, resources that would otherwise have been spent in treating malaria are put into other uses that enhance productivity such as schooling or farm investments.

It should be noted that the reduction in growth rate associated with malaria in Kenya in the 1980s is likely to be unreliable because it is based on macroeconometric estimates of the malaria burden for the whole of Sub-Saharan Africa. In addition to showing the magnitude of the loss in growth rate attributable to malaria, macroeconometric studies show that nearly ten per cent of GDP of African countries is lost to malaria annually (Gallup and Sachs, 1998). However, losses obtained using microeconomic methods (mainly the cost of illness approach) are generally smaller, and are in the order of 0.6–1 per cent of GDP (Ettling and Shepard, 1991; Malaney, 2000). In view of these malaria-related income losses, absolute poverty in Africa can be substantially reduced by controlling malaria in the region.

Even though the macroeconometric analysis shows that the economic burden of malaria in Africa is immense (Gallup and Sachs, 2000) and the estimates from micro, non-regression approaches are modest but significant (Ettling and Shepard, 1991), the few microeconometric studies available show little or no impact (Audibert, 1986; Wang'ombe and Mwabu, 1993).

What accounts for differences in macro-and micro-level economic burdens of malaria? The burden based on macro-evidence tends to be large because it captures negative externalities of malarial illnesses. For example, when farmers are unable to produce commercial food crops, preferring instead to produce subsistence crops such as cassava (because of the prevailing pattern of malaria prevalence), the nutritional effects of high food prices in urban areas and the associated productivity effects, are captured in a macro-level measurement of malaria burden. However, these effects are ignored at the micro-level.

Furthermore, although substitution of tasks within a household tends to reduce malaria burden at the household level in the short-run, it also tends to increase it in the long run, to the extent that it works against human capital formation by withdrawing children from school. Macro-level measurement of malaria burden takes into account both of these effects, whereas, the micro-level burden reflects only the short-run effect. Finally, in micro-based measurements of malaria burdens, e.g. those based on willingness to pay approach, the results tend to suffer from strategic and hypothetical biases, which are typically absent in macroeconometric studies (Okorosobo, 2000).

This chapter re-examines economic effects of malaria at the individual level in Kenya using a large household data set collected by the Central Bureau of Statistics, Ministry of Finance and Planning. Contrary to earlier microeconomic studies (based on limited data), we find large, negative economic effects of malaria at the micro level. In section two of the chapter, we depict the magnitude of malaria prevalence in Kenya by regions. In section three, we present the analytical framework and data sources. Simple, but important equations for measuring economic impacts of malaria are derived and interpreted. Section four is devoted to a presentation of regression results, which we discuss in Section five. The conclusion and suggestions for further research are in section six.

3.1 Malaria in Kenya

The magnitude of the malaria problem in a community can be measured in several ways. The most commonly and easily understood measure of malaria burden is the incidence rate of the disease in the population. Over 70 seventy per cent of the Kenyan population suffers from malaria infection at some point during the year. The disease is most common and dangerous among children and pregnant women. The prevalence of malaria in Kenya is highest in Western, Nyanza and Coast Provinces and has remained quite stable over time (Appendix Table 3.A1).

Malaria mortality is another measure of malaria burden in a community. Malaria specific mortality in Kenya (and Africa in general) is quite high relative to mortality from other diseases and from malaria in other regions (World Bank, 1993).

Another measure of the magnitude of malaria in the community is the intensity of the disease. Malaria intensity is measured by the parasite ratio of infection in the population. The parasite ratio is the percentage of children with detectable malaria *parasitaemia* in a given population.

Table 3.1 Median malaria *parasitaemia* rate in Kenyan children in selected study sites, 1998 (range of the ratios in parentheses)

Study Area (by Province and District)	Number of Study Sites	Parasite Ratios
Rift Valley Province		
Baringo	42	16.2 (3.1-48.9)
Kajiado	20	11.7 (2.2-21.2)
Turkana	27	24.2 (18.3-31.0)
Nandi	26	33.0 (3.0-91.0)
Narok	28	54.2
West Pokot	20	4.7 (3-65.0)
Western Province		
Bungoma	25	64.1 (32.1-84.0)
Busia	15	39.6 (11.7-47.2)
Kakamega	27	25.8 (14.6-77.8)
Vihiga	14	39.8 (33.6-46.0)

Continued

Table 3.1 *(continued)*

Study Area (by Province and District)	Number of Study Sites	Parasite Ratios
Coast Province		
Kwale	25	32.3 (12.7-64.4)
Kilifi	35	31.8 (4.5-75.1)
Lamu	9	8.5 (2.1-21.1)
Mombasa	12	21.2 (5.9-49.5)
Taita Taveta	16	20.2 (2.4-30.2)
Tana River	18	26.2 (3.8-73.5)
Nyanza Province		
Homa Bay	35	52.1 (24.8-78.8)
Kisii	25	66.1 (4.5-72.4)
Kisumu	27	58.7 (7.8-84.0)
Migori	28	37.3 (9.7-71.9)
Siaya	31	63.5 (60.5-94.5)
Eastern Province		
Embu	20	12.4 (10.3-14.4)
Kitui	35	20.9 (12.7-49.1)
Machakos	22	12.0 (0.0-44.4)
Makueni	21	20.0 (1.7-48.3)
Meru	39	0.4 (0.0-45.3)
Central Province		
Nyeri	30	0.0
Kiambu	29	17.4
Kirinyaga	17	2.6 (2.5-5.4)
All districts	1085	33.2(0.0-94.5)

Source: Omumbo *et al.*, (1998).

This parasite ratio is used to classify populations according to the extent they have been exposed to malaria. That is, according to whether intensity of malaria transmission (endemicity) in the population is *hypo*, *meso*, *hyper* or *holo*. Malaria transmission is an important determinant of the outcome of malaria infection and is key in determining the effectiveness of specific control measures. Table 3.1 shows median parasite ratios from selected study sites in Kenya.

Table 3.1 shows that *parasitaemia* rates in children vary widely in Kenya with prevalence of malaria being particularly high in Kisii, Siaya, Bungoma and Homa Bay. Low rates of malaria *parasitaemia* occur in Nyeri, Meru and Kirinyaga. Furthermore, as indicated by range values of *parasitaemia* rates, there is high variance of malaria prevalence within districts. The information in table 3.1 is valuable because in addition to indicating the pattern of provincial occurrence of malaria in the country, it also shows its intensity and variability within a district.

Table 3.1 suggests that the effects of malaria on production and incomes differ by regions, which further suggests that measures to control malaria and to mitigate its impact, should not be uniform throughout the country. Factors specific to regions, apart from endemicity, which may generate differences in economic effects of malaria in the country include health care seeking behavior, which in some instances is a cause and a consequence of drug resistance of particular strains of malaria (Musonda and Mangani; this volume). Other sources of differences in economic burdens of malaria include local economic activities, unemployment rate, and the spread and depth of poverty. High rates of unemployment, (that are conducive to substitution of tasks within a household) for example would tend to be associated with low economic burdens of malaria that are derived from household surveys. Furthermore, malaria burdens that are similarly derived, would be low in poor regions simply because the opportunity cost of the labor time of the poor people is low. To keep the study manageable, only a few of these determinants of malaria burden will be pursued in detail.

3.2 Model and Data

3.2.1 Preliminaries

The economic burden of malaria is defined here as the total loss in per capita household income or production associated with malaria morbidity and mortality. Although malaria is a source of much pain and suffering, we concentrate only on measurable economic damage due to malaria. The economic burden of malaria can be derived from estimates of a production function or its analog following the practice in macroeconometric literature (Gallup and Sachs, 2000; McCarthy *et al.,* 2000).

We start by elucidating the micro-economic context in which the measurement of the malaria burden is conducted. It is often analytically convenient to locate theoretical microeconomic analysis at the household level, even when the attendant empirical analysis is at the individual level. This is accomplished by assuming that the household head is a representative household member. The representative household member assumption yields the unitary model of household behavior, in which all household members share a common preference, which is typically maximized by the head. The "representativeness" assumption of course is an analytic device used to eliminate differences in purpose within a household so that diverse individuals who live in the same compound or who happen to pool livelihood resources despite being in different compounds, can act in unison in achieving their identical goals (Strauss and Thomas, 1998).

In our case, both the theoretical and empirical analyzes are at the individual level. Thus, the concept of a head, which is an institutional innovation for managing conflict within a household or a group, is unnecessary, as the focus is on one self-interested person. That is, there is no opportunity for conflicting preferences. However, the various individuals being studied differ in personal and other characteristics. For example, children and adults differ in their abilities to perform farm work and to earn wage incomes. Because of this difference in natural abilities, even after controlling for their health status, farm and non-farm productivities of adults and children would differ. If one does not control for this ability differential, production and income effects of health status and ability cannot be disentangled. As already noted, measurement of production effects of diseases is also complicated by possibilities for intra-household work substitutions and consumption smoothing strategies of households.

In the empirical analysis, we use the concept of "adult equivalence" to standardize production and incomes of individuals. That is, on average, each individual in a household is by construction the same as any other in terms of the ability to generate output or wage income, because all individuals are equivalent to a reference adult (Deaton, 1980). We used the procedure in Foster, Greer and Thorbecke (1984) to compute adult equivalents for each household. For example, if a household has three adults, that household has three adult equivalent units (1 adult is equal to 1 adult unit). On the other hand, if a household has three adults and two children, age five to nine years, it has four adult equivalent units (1 child is approximately equal to 0.6 of an adult based on nutritional requirements criteria).

However, differences in non-ability characteristics of individuals such as education and sex, and in household backgrounds such as household size, resource endowments and residence location, generate variations in average productivities of individuals across households. In contrast to the literature in this area (Strauss and Thomas, 1998), we do not deal with endogeneity of some of the variables in the estimating equations, particularly, health status (malaria morbidity) or household size due to data limitations.

3.2.2 Estimating equations

Since the purpose of this chapter is to measure the impact of malaria on farm output, wage incomes and household welfare generally, we estimate respectively, farm production functions, wage functions and household expenditure functions. We use household expenditure as a proxy for household permanent income. The general functional forms of the estimating equations are as follows:

$$Q = f(K, L, X, M) \quad (1)$$

$$W = g(S, Z, M) \quad (2)$$

$$Y = h(S, V, M) \quad (3)$$

where

Q = Quantity of agricultural output per adult equivalent in a given crop season;

W = Monthly earnings in Kenya shillings;
S = Years of schooling;
K = Household landholding per adult equivalent;
L = Household size;
X = A matrix of covariates (e.g. age, sex, residence location, interaction terms);
Z = A matrix of covariates (e.g. job experience, sex, residence location, interaction terms);
V = A matrix of covariates (e.g. age, household size, sex, residence location).
M = Malaria morbidity; M is malaria prevalence at the household level (the percentage of household members with malaria), or dummy variable indicating whether an individual has malaria or not.

We estimated various versions and specifications of the above three equations using household data. One of the innovations in the estimations concerns interaction of the malaria variable with education variable to assess the extent to which education alters the effect of illness (malaria) on household income or production. Although this practice of interacting variables is common in the general econometric literature, the institutional basis for it has, until recently (Fosu, 2001, 2002) been far from clear. To clarify the issue involved, consider the following simple linear specification of a farm production function.

$$Q = \alpha + \beta M + \varepsilon \quad \text{..} \quad (4)$$

where

Q is output per adult equivalent and β is the effect of malaria on average productivity of agricultural labor, α is a constant term, and ε is the usual disturbance term.

Equation (4) states a relationship between farm production and epidemiological environment. Since β is assumed to be negative, the equation states that the epidemiological environment (proxied by malaria) exerts a negative impact on farm production. Thus, without institutions that affect this impact, malaria will always reduce farm production. An example of such an institution is an education system that equips workers with knowledge about malaria prevention and treatment, in addition to increasing their productive skills. Thus, such an institution can affect farm production directly and/or by changing the size of β. The education system has the power to affect production directly because it enhances productivity of workers. The system can change the size of β by favorably altering the behavior of individuals towards malaria prevention and treatment, thus reducing the intensity of malaria.

In this case, a given malaria prevalence rate of a less intensive malaria infection would be associated with a smaller β than the same prevalence rate of a more intensive malaria infection. In that hypothetical case, education mitigates the impact of malaria on production. Education can also mitigate the effect of malaria on production and incomes by making workers more productive so that a given malaria prevalence rate has a bigger negative impact on production among less educated than among more educated workers. This hypothesis rests on the assumption that sick individuals continue to work after contracting malaria. The less educated workers who get malaria suffer greater production losses relative to the more educated workers because they have less human capital. However, if both types of workers miss work because of malaria illness, the disease burden is higher among the more educated workers because the opportunity cost of their time is higher.

There may be contexts in which the negative impact of malaria on production can be worsened by education. This can occur if the schooling environment reduces malaria immunity of workers so that the more educated workers tend to have greater intensity of malaria infections than the less educated. Because of the above considerations, the a priori sign of the coefficient on the interaction variable (education x malaria) is indeterminate. To fix ideas, we include an education variable in Equation (4) and rewrite it as follows.

$$Q = \alpha + \beta M + \delta (M \bullet S) + \gamma S + \varepsilon \quad \text{.................} \quad (4)$$

From expression (4), the production environment without malaria is described by the formula:

$$Q = \alpha + \gamma S \quad \text{..} \quad 5(a)$$

Similarly, the production environment with malaria (M=1) is described by the expression:

$$Q = (\alpha + \beta) + (\delta + \gamma)S \quad \text{.............................. 5(b)}$$

In Equation (5a), farm production is accounted for by the institutional factor, S (education investment), and by the omitted variables such as land and labor inputs which can easily be included in the equation.

In Equation (5b), the term (δS) either reduces or increases the absolute impact (β) of malaria on production. Mitigation occurs when δ is positive, and attenuation can occur (but rarely) when δ is negative. Similarly, ($\alpha+\beta$) is the extent of the downward shift in farm production function due to the negative effects of malaria on total factor productivity, α. Notice that production is always higher under (5a) than under (5b), even when in 5(b), the term (δS) is positive, i.e. the parameter, δ is positive. See Fosu (1992) for a similar econometric analysis in a different context.

If in Equation (4), Q is in log form and M is a dummy, the economic burden of malaria, Ψ, can be computed as:

$$\Psi = \{\exp(\beta) - 1.0\} \quad \text{.................................... (6a)}$$

In equation (6a), Ψ represents the percentage decline in household production or income due to malaria. (A common error in using expression (6a) is to fail to take into account the "negative sign" of the parameter β). The economic loss due to other diseases can be computed similarly. If in Equation (4), both Q and M are in *log form,* it is easily checked that the expression for the economic loss, λ is:

$$\lambda = (\partial Q / \partial M) = (Q/M) \bullet \beta \quad \text{................................ (6b)}$$

where,

β is the elasticity of production or income, Q, with respect to malaria prevalence, M. It is the economic burden of malaria expressed in percentage form, and Q and M are sample means. The economic loss in levels, λ, is the reduction in household production or income resulting from a unit increase in malaria prevalence at the household level. The parameter, λ, is always expressed in units in which Q is measured, e.g., kilograms in the case of farm output. Notice from Equation (6b) that the elasticity term,

$\beta = \lambda \cdot (M/Q)$. If in Equation (4), Q is in log form, and M is in levels, we have the following slight rearrangement of the preceding formula:

$$\beta = (\lambda/Q) \bullet M \quad \text{(6c)}$$

where, the quantity, (λ/Q), is known from regression results, and M is available from sample means.

3.2.3 Data

We estimated various versions of Equations (1–3) using different econometric methods with household data from the Central Bureau of Statistics, Ministry of Finance and Planning. The data come from a national probability sample of 10,857 households comprising 59,183 individuals. The data were collected from census-based enumeration clusters in all Kenyan provinces and districts. The data from the survey contains detailed information about household and individual characteristics, farm production, wage incomes, educational attainment, household expenditure and asset portfolios of households (Republic of Kenya, 1996, Mwabu *et al.*, 2000).

The analytic samples used for estimation were derived from the full probability sample of 59,183 individuals. Three steps were undertaken to construct the analytic samples. The first step entailed merging individual level data sets with data sets containing household characteristics. That is, individuals were matched with relevant characteristics of their own households. The second step required placing restrictions on merged data sets to create final analytic samples, and constructing proxy variables for malaria. Two indicators of malaria were constructed: a dummy variable showing whether or not an individual had reported having suffered from a malaria attack two weeks before the survey, and a continuous variable showing the proportion of household members who had contracted malaria during the same period. The dummy measure is an indicator variable showing a malaria episode at an individual level, while the continuous variable shows the prevalence of malaria (and possibly its intensity) in a household to which an individual lives. A dummy variable showing episodes of other diseases within a household was also constructed. The assessment of malaria on production, incomes and wages was conducted controlling for effects of other diseases. The assessment was done using ordinary least squares (OLS) and least absolute deviations (LAD) regression methods.

3.3 Results

We present OLS and median regression results regarding effects of malaria on crop production, wages and total household income (proxied by total household expenditure). The effects of malaria are measured controlling for other covariates of interest. We start by discussing results on crop production. The OLS and Median regression results are presented together to facilitate assessment of sensitivity of results to estimation methods, and to changes in the specification of models and measurement of malaria.

Table 3.2 Dependent variable: log crop output in long rains (malaria = prevalence rate)

Variables	OLS Regression		Median Regression	
	Parameter Estimates	*t*-ratios	Parameter Estimates	Bootstrap *t*-ratios
Proportion of Household Members Sick with Malaria Two Weeks Prior to the Survey	-.627*	-5.45	-.689*	-4.33
Proportion of Members Ill with Other Diseases (Proportion *Not Ill* is the Omitted Variable)	-.518*	-3.98	-.334*	-1.93
Log Years of Schooling	.074	1.12	.023	.19
Log Household Land Holding Per Adult Equivalent	.392*	14.45	.336*	6.57
Log Age	.164*	5.94	.262*	6.53
Log Household Size	-.758*	-11.99	-.869*	-.12.38
Residence (1 = Rural; 0 = Urban)	.077	.68	.132	-1.72
Sex (1 = Male; 0 = Female)	.216*	4.70	.304*	5.76
Constant	3.598*	16.49	3.902*	18.45
Adj R-Squared (Pseudo R-Squared)	0.077		0.043	
Sample Size	7602			

* Statistically significant at the 5% level.

Source: Own calculations based on Welfare Monitoring Household Survey, 1994.

3.3.1 Effects of malaria on crop production

The results for this sub-section are in tables 3.2–3.5. Tables 3.2 and 3.3 show effects of malaria on crop production in long and short rains, with the malaria variable being defined as the household level malaria prevalence rate (i.e. proportion of household members infected with malaria two weeks prior to the survey). Tables 3.2–3.4 show that the effect of malaria illness on crop production is negative and statistically significant. This finding persists irrespective of the estimation method, and irrespective of whether malaria illness is proxied by its prevalence within a household (a continuous

Table 3.3 Dependent variable: log crop output in short & long rains (malaria = prevalence rate)

Variables	OLS Regression		Median Regression	
	Parameter Estimates	*t*-ratios	Parameter Estimates	Bootstrap *t*-ratios
Proportion of Household Members Sick with Malaria Two Weeks Prior to the Survey	-.399*	-3.68	-.516*	-3.63
Proportion of Members Ill with Other Diseases (Proportion *Not Ill* is the Omitted Variable)	-.325*	-2.69	-.195	-1.06
Log Years of Schooling	.044	.72	-.015	-.22
Log Household Land Holding in Acres per Adult Equivalent	.371*	15.21	.329*	9.84
Log Age	.124*	4.77	.213*	6.16
Log Household Size	.568*	10.06	.417*	8.26
Residence (1 = Rural; 0 = Urban)	.027	.25	-.094	.89
Sex (1 = Male; 0 = Female)	.188*	4.44	.227*	4.02
Constant	3.127*	15.53	3.502*	19.75
Adj R-Squared (Pseudo R-Squared)	0.037		0.017	
Sample Size	8834			

* Statistically significant at the 5% level.

Source: Own calculations based on Welfare Monitoring Household Survey, 1994.

variable), or by identification of a household member afflicted by the disease (a dichotomous variable).

Table 3.2 shows that malaria reduces crop output more relative to other diseases. Looking at the median regression estimates (which are insensitive to data outliers), it can be seen that the negative production effect of malaria is more than twice the effect of other diseases (Tables 3.2 and 3.3). In table 3.4, where malaria is defined as dummy, its negative production effect is much larger than that of other diseases.

Tables 3.2 and 3.3 show that other statistically important determinants of crop production include gender, experience (proxied by age), land holding and household size. In particular crop production rises with land holding per adult equivalent and with experience (age minus six minus years of schooling). On average, output per adult equivalent is higher among men than women and is unaffected by whether the family head lives in a rural or urban area. Effects of family size on farm output are mixed, and no statistically significant effect of years of schooling on farm output is detectable from data.

The OLS regression in table 3.4 is based on a sub-sample consisting of healthy individuals and individuals afflicted with malaria. Thus, the coefficient on malaria dummy shows the extent to which farm output is lower among malaria sufferers relative to farm output of healthy individuals. In contrast, the median regression is estimated with a sub-sample of individuals who had suffered from both malaria and other diseases two weeks before the survey date, pooled with a sub-sample of healthy individuals. This was done to assess how "being ill" affects farm output. Thus, the coefficient on disease dummy in the LAD regression shows the magnitude by which the log of farm output of ill individuals falls below that of healthy individuals.

The OLS results indicate that individuals afflicted with malaria are less productive relative to people afflicted with other diseases. The same result is generated by the median regression. However, although other diseases also reduce output, their effect is statistically insignificant. Furthermore, the effect of malaria in the OLS regression is much larger than in the median regression. Even though these magnitudes are not comparable (because the sample sizes differ), the comparatively large effect in the median regression should be noted. The smaller coefficients in the OLS regression are probably accounted for by substitution of tasks between sick and healthy individuals. Also noteworthy from the OLS regression, is the positive but insignificant effect of interaction of schooling with malaria. Generally, the effect of education on farm output is statistically insignificant in all the regressions reported in the above tables.

Table 3.4 Dependent variable: log crop output in long rains (malaria = 1 if individual had malaria and 0 if other diseases)

Variables	OLS Regression		Median Regression	
	Parameter Estimates	*t*-ratios	Parameter Estimates	Bootstrap *t*-ratios
Malaria = 1 if individual had malaria and = 0 if had other diseases	-.107*	-2.90	-.237*	-2.73
Disease = 1 if malaria and other diseases (*healthy* individuals are the comparison group)	–	–	-.056	-.72
Log Years of Schooling	.029*	2.25	-.320	-.27
Log Household Land Holding Per Adult Equivalent	.119*	10.02	.375	.03
Log Age	.084*	7.71	-.168	-.06
Log Household Size	-.758*	-23.89	.564*	12.72
Residence (1 = Rural; 0 = Urban)	-.127	-1.85	-.133	1.74
Sex (1 = Male; 0 = Female)	.141*	6.50	–	–
Malaria x Years of Schooling	.029	.91	–	–
Constant	3.840*	43.66	3.502*	19.75
Adj R-Squared (Pseudo R-Squared)	0.026		0.037	
Sample Size	33054		7602	

* Statistically significant at the 5% level.
Source: Own calculations based on Welfare Monitoring Household Survey, 1994.

3.3.2 Effects of malaria on wages

Table 3.5 depicts effects of malaria on monthly wage incomes in a sample of sick and healthy individuals. The estimated Mincerian log wage function shows very small returns to schooling; 1.3 per cent in the OLS regression and 1.7 per cent in the Median regression. The coefficients of interactions of malaria with schooling are positive but insignificant in both regressions. The effects of malaria on wages are negative, as expected, but statistically insignificant. The positive coefficient on the interaction of malaria with schooling suggests that education mitigates the negative production effects of malaria. Other notable results from the table include higher log wages for men than for women, and in urban than in rural areas.

Table 3.5 Dependent variable: log monthly wage (malaria = 1 if individual had malaria and 0 if other disease)

Variables	OLS Regression		Median Regression	
	Parameter Estimates	***t*-ratios**	**Parameter Estimates**	**Bootstrap *t*-ratios**
Malaria = 1 if individual had malaria and = 0 if had other diseases (*other* diseases omitted)	-.160	-1.81	-.169	-1.09
Log Years of Schooling	.013	.093	.017	1.62
Log Years of Job Experience	.473*	2.17	.719*	2.16
Log Experienced Squared	-.071	-1.54	.122	-1.85
Residence (1 = Rural; 0 = Urban)	-.1.711*	-14.65	-.1.750*	-16.75
Sex (1 = Male; 0 = Female)	1.579*	20.29	1.586*	11.32
Malaria x Log Years of Schooling	.024	1.27	.019	.97
Constant	4.729*	15.51	4.729*	14.57
Adj R-Squared (Pseudo R-Squared)	0.118		0.069	
Sample Size	5550		5550	

* Statistically significant at the 5% level.

Source: Own calculations based on Welfare Monitoring Household Survey, 1994.

The results in table 3.5 are based on a sub-sample of workers with malaria or other illness. Thus the coefficient on malaria shows the effect of malaria on wages relative to the effect of other diseases. The statistical insignificance of malaria coefficient in table 3.5 is probably a reflection of institutions in labor markets that insulate workers' wages from effects of illnesses. Such institutions could include paid sick-off from work, a wage contract that is difficult to change because of illness, and a remuneration scheme unrelated to productivity. Furthermore, availability of quality health services for individuals with wage employment can help restore health before the adverse productivity effects of illness set in.

3.3.3 Effects of malaria on per capita household expenditure

The results in table 3.6 are obtained from a sub-sample of ill individuals. That is, healthy individuals were excluded from the sample to create an analytic sub-sample comprising individuals with malaria and other diseases. In such a sub-sample, substitution of tasks among individuals, which tends to show "perverse" or no effects of malaria on production is weakened, because the sample consists of ill individuals only. In a sample consisting of healthy and sick individuals, regression coefficients on malaria dummies were occasionally positive, probably because ill individuals were substituted by more productive workers. Since the aim of the study was to estimate effects of illness on production (per capita income), it was desirable to control for effects of all other factors, including the intra-household exchange of tasks. Effects of such exchanges on per capita income are best mitigated, in this case, by a sample consisting of ill individuals where opportunities for exchange of tasks are limited. Unfortunately, it is necessary in this case to make the strong assumption that the severity of illness is the same across individuals.

The coefficient on malaria in table 3.6 shows the impact of malaria on household income relative to other diseases, without directly controlling for per capita income of healthy individuals in a regression equation. (However, note that the method of sample construction indirectly controls for per capita income of healthy individuals). The results in table 3.6 are similar to those presented in previous tables. Income losses from malaria are greater than losses from other diseases.

The implication here is that malaria impairs work ability more relative to other diseases. Since ability to work is compromised by any disease, the results strongly suggest that sick people have lower incomes than healthy people. In particular, an individual's income is lower in the event of malaria episode than in the event of any other disease. As in previous tables, the coefficient on interaction of malaria with schooling mitigates the impact of malaria, but caution is necessary because the coefficient lacks statistical significance.

Table 3.6 Dependent variable: log total household expenditure per month (malaria = 1 if individual had malaria and 0 if other disease)

Variables	OLS Regression		Median Regression	
	Parameter Estimates	*t*-ratios	Parameter Estimates	Bootstrap *t*-ratios
Malaria = 1 if individual had malaria and = 0 if had other diseases (*other* diseases omitted)	-.017	-.98	-.495	-1.79
Log Years of Schooling	.038*	3.15	-.071	-.1.34
Log Household Land Holding Per Adult Equivalent	.094*	11.36	.104*	4.71
Log Age	-.072*	-11.15	-.010	-.86
Log Household Size	-.679*	-32.56	.505*	16.93
Residence (1 = Rural; 0 = Urban)	-.507*	-13.44	-.752*	-8.88
Sex (1 = Male; 0 = Female)	-.008	.52	.001	.02
Malaria x Years of Schooling	-.028	-1.74	.202	1.55
Constant	10.43*	202.2	11.01*	58.26
Adj R-Squared (Pseudo R-Squared)	0.121		0.109	
Sample Size	10142		2484	

* Statistically significant at the 5% level.

Source: Own calculations based on Welfare Monitoring Household Survey, 1994.

Table 3.7 The economic burden of malaria in Kenya, 1994

Type of Production or Income Reduced by Malaria	Percentage by which Malaria Reduces Production or Income (Economic Burden of Malaria)	
	OLS Estimates	LAD Estimates
Monthly Wages	14.79%	15.55%
Crop Production (Long Rains)	10.15%	21.10%
Monthly Household Income per Capita	1.69%	39.04%

Source: Own calculations based on Tables 3.4–3.6.

3.4 Summarizing Economic Effects of Malaria

We use expression 6(a) and tables 3.4–3.6 to compute economic effects of malaria. From table 3.7, it can be seen that in 1994, malaria reduced wage incomes by fifteen to sixteen per cent relative to other diseases, whose effect has been normalized to zero in order to identify the effect of malaria. Notice that because of this normalization, the negative coefficient on malaria dummy is the magnitude by which malaria reduces wages or output over and above the reduction imposed by other diseases. Thus, the figures shown in table 3.7 are the benefits of malaria eradication (not reduction).

In 1994, crop production fell by anywhere from ten to twenty one per cent due to malaria, depending on the estimation method used to derive this impact. The losses in household income due to malaria vary substantially depending on the estimation method used to derive them. The losses associated with the OLS method are minimal, amounting to 1.7 per cent; while the losses obtained with the LAD method are quite large, thirty nine per cent. These estimates have been obtained assuming that effects of interaction terms in the regression equations do not matter, which is a fair assumption given their statistical insignificance.

In general, the economic losses due to malaria in table 3.7 are smaller than the losses reported in macroeconometric literature on the impact of malaria on national incomes and economic growth in Africa. Gallup and Sachs

(2000) for example report that African incomes are only one-third of incomes of countries without malaria. That is, national incomes in Africa are only one-third of the incomes the continent would be enjoying if it were free from malaria. The very high LAD estimate of the loss in household income associated with malaria is certainly consistent with macroeconomic evidence. However, this is a very preliminary figure because there are many variables that have not been fully controlled for in its estimation. Furthermore, there are a number of econometric issues to be addressed, particularly the endogeneity of malaria illness before the estimate can be taken seriously. Income and production losses of ten to twenty one per cent also find some support in macroeconomic literature on economic burden of malaria.

The elasticities reported in table 3.8 were obtained using expression 6(c.) in the text, and the results in tables 3.2 and 3.3 plus the sample statistics in Appendix 3.A1 (i.e., the means for malaria and other diseases). Table 3.8 shows that farm output is inelastic with respect to prevalence of malaria and other diseases. Taking LAD figures as the more reliable estimates, a ten per cent increase in malaria prevalence rate, for example, is associated with a three per cent mean reduction in farm output. The corresponding elasticity for other diseases combined is 1.3 per cent, which is much smaller than the elasticity for malaria.

The relatively large economic burden of malaria partly arises from the widespread nature of the disease. As can be seen from appendix table 3.A1, malaria alone constituted fifty per cent of self reported morbidity in 1994. Recent epidemiological data shows that malaria prevalence in Kenya is not only on the increase, but the disease has become resistant to commonly used drugs, a fact that is likely to accelerate its prevalence in the future. There is urgency therefore, in controlling the spread of the disease to avoid further economic losses associated with it.

3.5 Discussion

It is important to distinguish between the difference between tables 3.7 and 3.8. Table 3.7 shows incomes and farm output in a malarial environment relative to a situation without malaria. Thus, as already noted, the figures in table 3.7 are percentages by which incomes and farm output would

Table 3.8 Elasticities of farm outputs with respect to malaria and other diseases

Season	Elasticity of Farm Production with Respect to:			
	Malaria		Other Diseases	
	OLS Estimates	LAD Estimates	OLS Estimates	LAD Estimates
Long Rains	-.315	-.346	-.258	-.166
Short and Long Rains	-.200	-.257	-.162	-.097
Mean	-.257	-.302	-.210	-.129

Source: Own calculations based on Tables 2 and 3.

increase if malaria were to be *eliminated.* For example, eradication of malaria would increase wage incomes by fifteen to sixteen per cent. In other words, the table shows economic effects of a quantum change in a malarial environment.

In contrast, table 3.8 shows economic benefits of marginal changes in malarial environment. It depicts economic benefits of small reductions in malaria prevalence. For example, a one per cent reduction in malaria prevalence would increase farm production in the long rains by 0.346 per cent (Table 3.8, LAD estimate).

To see clearly the connection between tables 3.7 and 3.8, we first focus attention on tables 3.2 and 3.7. We start by noting that the economic effect of a quantum change in malaria environment (Table 3.7) is equivalent to the effect of reducing malaria prevalence from its present level (50.2%, see Table 3.A1) to zero per cent. Since the response of the log of farm output in the long rains to a level percentage change in malaria prevalence is –.689 (Table 3.2, LAD estimate), reducing malaria prevalence from .502 to zero would increase farm output (labor productivity) by (–.689*–.502) = 34.6 per cent. Although smaller, this is generally within the range depicted by the LAD estimate (21.1%) of the economic burden of malaria (Table 3.7). In table 3.7, the LAD estimate indicates that farm output would be 21.1 per cent higher in a malaria free environment.

Based on LAD estimates, eradication of other diseases (reducing their prevalence from 48.9 per cent to zero per cent) would increase farm output during the long rains season by 16.6 per cent (=–.334*–.498). Thus, eradication of malaria and other diseases would increase farm production during the long rains by 51.22 per cent. Since poverty incidence in Kenya is highest in the agricultural sector, a disease control program is an important component of a poverty reduction strategy.

The above discussion shows that multiplication of coefficients on disease prevalence in table 3.2 with sample prevalence rates in table 3.A1 yields the elasticity figures in table 3.8. At this point, connecting tables 3.7 and 3.8 involves a trivial calculation. As already noted, table 3.8 shows malaria prevalence elasticities of outputs and incomes. However, notice that malaria eradication (reducing malaria prevalence from 50.2 per cent to zero per cent involves a "proportional" (as opposed to a "level") reduction in malaria prevalence of 100 per cent =[–.502/.502)*100]. It is easily checked that malaria eradication (starting from any level), involves a 100 per cent reduction in malaria prevalence.

Thus, multiplication of elasticities in table 3.8 with "proportional" percentage reduction in malaria prevalence, following malaria eradication, yields the corresponding percentage increases in output and incomes. The multiplication is a trivial calculation because it only involves moving the decimal point in each entry in table 3.8 two places to the right. Hence, percentage increases in incomes or outputs following malaria eradication (as in Table 3.7) are "immediately" available from disease prevalence elasticities (as in Table 3.8). For example, the elasticity of farm output with respect to malaria prevalence of (.346) in table 3.8 indicates that malaria eradication would increase output by 34.6 per cent (the corresponding figure in Table 3.7 is 21.1 per cent). Focusing attention on production effects of malaria in the long rains, a comparison of tables 3.7 and 3.8 shows that in this data set, disease burdens computed when malaria is defined as a discrete variable (Table 3.7) are smaller than those derived when malaria is defined as a continuous variable (Table 3.8).

We note in passing that an increase in malaria prevalence from zero per cent to any positive number involves infinitely large percentage reductions in incomes. Although this result follows mechanically from the definition of an elasticity, it has some application in the case of malaria. A non-localized modest increase in malaria incidence (from zero per cent level to say ten per cent), can quickly devastate a labor force that has no malaria immunity.

It should be pointed out that policy implications of the findings in tables 3.7 and 3.8 are overstated. Malaria eradication is no longer considered a feasible policy objective (Snow *et al.,* 1997) in health sectors. Instead, the objective of many governments (Kenya's included) in the health sector, is to control malaria to a tolerable level. Thus, during a given time period, only fractions of the benefits shown in tables 3.7 and 3.8 can be realized because malaria eradication is infeasible over the interval. Furthermore, since any reduction in malaria over time comes from several sources (including non-program sources), only fractions of the benefits associated with the reduction can be attributed to control programs.

Attribution of such benefits is not a simple task however. There is need to devise practical methods of assigning benefits of reductions in malaria incidence over time to specific control programs. There is also need to point out that the endogeneity of malaria has been ignored in the estimated models due to lack of proper instruments. As a result, it was not possible to obtain consistent estimates of the malaria burden. However, the results reported here provide some preliminary evidence of the economic burden of malaria at the household level, and point to rough orders of magnitude as to the benefits of controlling this disease.

3.6 Conclusion

Malaria afflicts a large number of people in Kenya. In addition to pain, anxiety and suffering that the disease causes, its economic burden is immense. Using the 1994 welfare monitoring data set, we have quantified the economic losses from malaria. Because of the adverse productivity effects of malaria, Kenyan wage incomes in 1994 were fifteen to sixteen per cent lower than they should have been in the absence of malaria. The reduction in farm output was even higher, in the order of ten to twenty one per cent. The toll of malaria on per capita income was nearly forty per cent, which is in the same order of magnitude as the losses reported in macroeconometric literature. In view of these losses, we find that an effective malaria control program in the country would increase household income considerably and help reduce poverty.

However, in order to design and implement such a strategy effectively, additional research is required in several areas. The first area of research relates to demand for malaria treatments. Information is required to inform policy on health care seeking behavior of malaria patients, including how such behavior is affected by economic and non-economic factors. Despite a large literature on awareness of causes of malaria (Rosenfield, *et al.*, 1981; Spencer, *et al.*, 1987), scanty econometric analysis exists on the determinants of malaria treatments (de Batolome and Vosti, 1995). As a consequence, scarcely little is known about quantitative effects of malaria control on health care seeking behavior and hence on possible outcomes of control measures. A similar analysis is needed on demand for preventive malaria services (see Kamgnia, this volume; Wang'ombe and Mwabu, 1993).

Another research area relates to cost-benefit analysis of malaria control strategies. Since an analysis such as the one undertaken in this chapter provides quantitative information as to benefits of malaria control measures, it is now possible to compute cost-benefit ratios of the available control measures. Such ratios should be invaluable in designing advocacy strategies for malaria control and in communicating to policy makers the benefits of investing in health more generally (Schultz, 1999). A third research area suggested by this chapter concerns the role institutions can play in mitigating impacts of malaria on incomes and farm production. Finally, there is need to examine *ex ante*, managerial constraints in the implementation of national malaria control programs.

References

Akin, J.S. *et al.*, (1986), "The Demand for Primary Health Care Services in the Bicol Region of the Philippines". *Economic Development and Cultural Change* 34: 755–782.

Arndt, C. and Lewis, J.D. (2000), "The Macro Implications of HIV/AIDS in South Africa: A Preliminary Assessment". *South African Journal of Economics* 68 (5): 856–887.

Audibert, M. (1986), "Agricultural Non-wage Production and Health Status: A Case Study in a Tropical Environment". *Journal of Development Economics* 24: 275–291.

De Bartolome, C.A.M. and Vosti, S.A. (1995), "Choosing Between Public and Private Health-Care: A Case Study of Malaria Treatment in Brazil". *Journal of Health Economics,* Vol. 14: 191–205.

Deaton, A. and Muellbauer, J. (1980), *Economics and Consumer Behavior.* Cambridge: Cambridge University Press.

Ettling, M.B. and Shepard, D.S. (1991), "The Economic Cost of Malaria in Rwanda". *Trop. Med. Parasitol.* 42 (Suppl. 1): 214–218.

Foster, J.E, Greer, J., and Thorbecke, E. (1984), "A Class of Decomposable Poverty Measures". *Econometrica* 52 (3): 761–766.

Gallup, J.L. and Sachs, J.D. (2000), "The Economic Burden of Malaria". Harvard University, Center for International Development, CID Working Paper, No. 52, July.

Fosu, A.K. (1992), "Political Instability and Economic Growth: Evidence from Sub-Saharan Africa". *Economic Development and Cultural Change*, 829–841.

Fosu, A.K. (2001), "Political Instability and Economic Growth in Developing Countries: Some Specification Empirics". *Economics Letters* Vol. 70: 289–294.

Fosu, A.K. (2002), "Transforming Economic Growth into Human Development in Sub-Saharan Africa: The Role of Elite Political Economy". *Oxford Development Studies* 30 (1): 9–19.

Kamgnia, B. (2007), "The Demand for Malaria Control Products and Services: Evidence from Yaounde, Cameroon", this volume.

Malaney, P. (2000), "The Microeconomic Burden of Malaria", Harvard University, CID Working Paper, Mimeo.

McCarthy, D.F., Wolf, H., Wu, Y. (1999), "Malaria and Growth", Department of Economics, Georgetown University, Mimeo.

Musonda, F. and Mangani, F. (2007), "The Distribution of Pharmaceutical Products and Malaria Control in Zambia", this Volume.

Mwabu, G., *et al.,* (2000), "Poverty in Kenya: Profiles and Determinants", AERC Report, Nairobi, Mimeo.

Okorosobo, T. (2000), "The Economic Burden of Malaria in Africa", Paper prepared for the Abuja Summit of Heads of State and Government, Abuja, Nigeria, April.

Omumbo, J., Ouma, J., Rapuoda, B., Craig, M.H., Le Sueur, D. and Snow, R.W. (1998), "Mapping Malaria Transmission Intensity Using Geographical Information Systems: An Example from Kenya". *Annals of Tropical Medicine and Parasitology*, Vol. 92, No. 1: 7–21.

Republic of Kenya (1996), *Kenya Welfare Monitoring Survey, 1994.* Nairobi: Central Bureau of Statistics, Ministry of Finance and Planning.

Rosenfield, P.L., Wistrand, C., and Runderman, A.P. (1981), "Social and Economic Research in UNDP-World Bank-WHO Special Program of Research and Training in Tropical Diseases". *Social Science and Medicine* 15A, No. 5: 529–538.

Shepard, D.S, Ettling, M.B., Brinkmann, U., and Sauerborn, R. (1991), "The Cost of Malaria in Africa". *Trop. Med. Parasitol.* 42 (Suppl. 1): 199–203.

Schultz, T. P. (1999), "Health and Schooling Investments in Africa". *Journal of Economic Perspectives* 13 (3): 67–88.

Snow, R.W., Omumbo, J.A., Lowe, B., Molyneux, C.S., Obiero, C.S., Palmer, J.O., Weber, A., Pinder, M.W. *et al.,* (1997), "Relation Between Severe Malaria Morbidity in Children and Level of *Plasmodium falciparum* Transmission in Africa". *Lancet,* I:1650–1654.

Spencer, H.C., *et al.,* (1987), "Community-based Malaria Control in Saradidi, Kenya". *Annals of Tropical Medicine*, Vol. 81 (Suppl. 1), 13–23.

Strauss, J. and Thomas, D. (1998), "Health, Nutrition and Development". *Journal of Economic Literature* 36 (2): 766–817.

Wang'ombe, J.K. and Mwabu, G. (1993), "Agricultural Land Use Patterns and Malaria Conditions in Kenya". *Social Science and Medicine,* Vol. 37, No. 9:1121–1130.

World Bank (1993), *World Development Report.* Oxford University Press.

Chapter 3 Appendix Table

Appendix Table 3.A1 Sample statistics for selected variables for sick individuals, 1994

Variable	Sample	Mean	Std Dev
Years of Job Experience	5,550	15.1	12.8
Experience Squared	5,550	226.8	163.8
Monthly Wages (Ksh)	13,727	246.8	1627.5
Crop Production in Long and Short Rains (Kg)	9,870	457.0	1944.7
Crop Production in Long Rains Per Adult Equivalent (Kg)	9,870	33.7	170.8
Crop Production in Short Rains Per Adult Equivalent (Kg)	9,870	104.5	600.7
Percentage Male	13,727	45.8%	49.8%
Percentage Ill With Malaria	13,727	50.2%	50.0%
Percentage Ill With Other Diseases	13,727	49.8%	50.0%
Monthly Expenditure Per Capita (Ksh)	13,727	19,723.0	16,269.0
Number of Adult Equivalents in a Household	13,727	3.73	1.89
Household Size	13,727	4.41	1.44
Age in Years	13,007	21.26	20.68
Land Holding Per Adult Equivalent (acres)	10,686	1.62	3.02
Percentage of Rural Individuals	13,727	87.3%	33.3%

Source: Own calculation based on welfare monitoring survey, 1994.

Chapter 4

The Economic Burden of Childhood Malaria in Nigeria

Olufunke A. Olagoke

4.0 Motivation and Purpose

For more than fifty years, the mantra of "one million annual deaths due to malaria" in Africa and elsewhere has been cited by scientists and journalists. Until recently, this estimate had generally gone unexamined with regard to its accuracy, clinical components, and economic implications. The most recent estimate indicates that at a minimum, between 700,000 and 2.7 million people die annually from malaria, and that over the last decade (1995–2005), seventy five per cent of them were African children. The new data shows that between 400 and 900 million acute febrile episodes occur annually in under-five children living in malaria-endemic regions of Africa. Reports also suggest that this number is likely to double by 2020 if effective control interventions are not implemented (MIM, 2001).

The burden of malaria may have so far been underestimated because most of the existing studies have regularly provided only quantitative evidence on the impact of a person's health on his or her own time allocation, productivity, profits and wage rate. The fact, however, is that not all costs of malaria attack are borne by the individual whose health is impaired. Within the household, malaria attack on one individual (especially a dependant) is likely to evoke resources adjustment by other persons in the household in which the illness occurs. For instance, family members allocate more time to children when they are ill. This time is often transferred from other productive activities performed in and out of the household system (Pitt and Rosenzweig, 1990).

Consideration for the total spectrum of the effect of malaria within the household system is essential in determining the connections between malaria and poverty within the household. Although linkage between malaria and poverty has severally been speculated, an exhaustive investigation of sources of linkage is still lacking and requires greater consideration. Although studies often mention an intimate connection between malaria and poverty across the globe, the direction and extent of causality is however still very controversial. Evidence (Weller, 1958) suggests that countries in the poorest continent are most affected by malaria.

Africa is in this category and she is highly impoverished. Mwabu (2001) reports that well over fifty per cent of the people living in the continent is in abject poverty and about the same proportion is periodically being afflicted by malaria all through their lifetime. The only parts of Africa currently free of malaria are the northern and southern extremes, which are the richer countries in the continent. Interestingly, beyond the African continent, India has the greatest number of poor people in the world, and also has a serious malaria crisis. Evidence from the Western Hemisphere also indicates that Haiti, which has the highest incidence of malaria, is the poorest country in that hemisphere (Gallup and Sachs, 2000).

Malaria remains a major source of retardation to economic growth. For example, average growth of income per capita from 1965 to 1990 for countries with severe malaria transmission was only 0.4 per cent per year, whereas economic growth for countries with fewer malaria incidences was 2.3 per cent per year, more than five times higher (Gallup and Sachs, 2001). In 1993, the World Bank estimates showed that not less than thirty five million future life-years would be lost yearly to malaria infection. Sub-Saharan Africa's (SSA) case is particularly pathetic. Malaria is holoendemic in the region, and it depresses the region's gross domestic product (GDP) by about twenty per cent after every fifteen years (African Summit on Roll Back Malaria, April, 2000). With the current trend in endemicity, severity and resistance to traditional first-line drugs, the physical and economic burden of malaria in SSA may be a lot higher.

At the micro-level, a study on Nigeria in the early 1990s estimated that malaria episode per adult a year was an average of three, while work days lost in the process was also an average of three days (Foster *et al.*, 1993).

More current evidence from a global perspective by McCarthy and Wolf (2000) indicates that a typical bout of malaria now lasts from about ten to fourteen days, with four to six days of near complete incapacitation, and recuperation periods of four to eight days, which are characterized by fatigues and weakness.

Malaria has direct impact on households' income, wealth, productivity, and labor market participation of both the sick and their caregivers. This effect has a further impact on aggregate economic growth. The disease affects welfare and growth in a number of dynamic ways. One, it retards inflow of human and physical investment by affecting international itinerant groups moving into malaria endemic areas. Two, malaria demobilizes economically active portion of populations in endemic areas, leading to loss of substantial man-hours due to complete incapacitation or partial activity during the sickness period. Three, incidence of malaria in children and pregnant women attracts the greatest burden; apart from direct effect on children substantial productive time and resources are lost by caregivers. There is also a growing concern about the spreading incidence of drug resistant malaria in the continent (Mosanya, 1997), which tends to require more intensive attention than ever before.

This chapter is motivated by the increasing number of children who attend clinics in Nigeria due to malaria incidence, and the magnitude of malaria problem in the country. The study focuses on hospital-based survey of malaria burden in children, their caregivers and the welfare of the households by analyzing the direct and indirect losses due to malaria and the distribution of the burden. It also investigates the connection between malaria and poverty at the household level, and estimates gains from adequate malaria management in Nigeria.

4.1 Socioeconomic and Demographic Context

4.1.1 Demographic and health profile

Nigeria is a republic of thirty seven States (including the Federal Capital Territory) lying on the West Coast of Africa with a land area of 923,708 square kilometers. The country has a total population of about 120 million people (projected from 1991 population census). About forty eight per cent of the population is under fifteen years of age; forty nine per cent falls between fifteen–sixty four years' strata and three per cent are above sixty five years. Adult literacy rate is about fifty seven per cent. About seventy per cent of the population lives in the rural areas and the rest in semi-urban, and urban areas. Even with only thirty per cent of the Nigerian population living in urban areas, the centers are mostly over-crowded, a factor which enhances the rate of malaria transmission and inhibits effective prevention efforts.

According to the Federal Ministry of Health (1994–1995), Nigerian population under the age of five years is about 7.3 million, while the annual growth rate of the country's total population is three per cent. Crude birth is forty three live births per 1,000, and crude death rate is five per 1000 population. Infant mortality rate is 114 per 1,000 live births; maternal mortality rate is 800 per 100,000 live births. Under five-mortality rate is 119 per 1,000 live births. Complete immunization before age one is just thirty seven per cent and under-five malnutrition rate is thirty six per cent.

Malaria's contribution to the health problems in Nigeria is quite significant. For instance, malaria accounts for thirty per cent of all childhood deaths. The disease is also responsible for about eleven per cent of maternal deaths and contributes considerably to adult morbidity every year (Pediatric Association of Nigeria, 1994; Binka, 2000; National Malaria Control Program Plan of Action, 1996–2001; WHO, 2000).

4.1.2 Malaria morbidity, mortality and poverty

Malaria transmission in Sub-Saharan Africa is the highest in the world. Malaria parasite is transmitted into human blood stream via the infected bite of female anopheles mosquito. *Plasmodium falciparum* is the most dominant parasite species causing malignant tertian malaria and is responsible for over ninety per cent of infections in Nigeria (Ekanem, 1997). Plasmodium falciparum is highly notorious for causing severe and complicated malaria, often leading to death. It also has a vast capacity to develop resistance to anti-malarial drugs (Ekanem, 1997).

As in many SSA countries, recorded infective mosquito bites per person is in thc neighborhood of 100 bites per year in many parts of Nigeria. The intensity and velocity of these infective bites lead to frequent morbidity, mortality and serious loss to individuals as well as the households, and on the aggregate, to the national economy. Perhaps the increasing losses at micro-level in malaria endemic countries like Nigeria make them some of the world's most impoverished (Gallup and Sachs 2000, World Health Organization 1999, McCarthy, Wolf and Wu, 2000).

A focused malaria prevention and control initiative is important in addressing rising morbidity, mortality, low productivity and poverty in Nigeria. Malaria is endemic throughout the country; it accounts for fifty per cent of outpatient consultation and about fifteen per cent of hospital admissions; and is among the top three causes of death in the country. Approximately, fifty per cent of the population experiences at least one malaria episode per year, although the annual average is as much as four bouts in Nigerian children (National Malaria Control Plan of Action, 1996–2001). The trend is rapidly increasing due to the current malaria resistance to first line anti-malarial drugs (WHO, 2000).

Existing data indicates that malaria is the most prevalent of all major tropical diseases in the country; the magnitude of incidence and death due to it are a multiple of all other tropical diseases put together. Available data on the reported incidence of major tropical diseases in Nigeria shows the dominance of malaria. Table 4.1 below presents reported incidences of malaria and other tropical diseases in Nigeria.

Calculations based on table 4.1 reveal that malaria is responsible for over ninety per cent of tropical disease incidences reported in Nigeria. The data suggest that malaria may be the largest contributor to total disease burden and productivity losses resulting from major diseases in the country.

Table 4.1 Reported incidence of tropical diseases in Nigeria (period average in '000)

Period	Filiaris	Onchocercariasis	Malaria	Schistosomiasis
1971-75	24.4	11	832	24
1976-80	25.8	8.4	1024.4	26.8
1981-85	17.6	7	1276.8	38.6
1986-90	8.2	2.8	1105	24.6
1991-95	12.2	4.6	1110.4	15.2

Source: Calculated from *FOS Statistical Bulletin* (Various Issues).

The table shows that reported cases of malaria are numerous while, all other tropical diseases put together are not as many. The above estimate, is however, a far cry from actual malaria incidence in Nigeria as unrecorded incidence is multiple of times higher (Mosanya, 1997).

The disease carries with it two categories of costs; morbidity and mortality costs. Malaria morbidity affects household's welfare (through families' allocation to treatment and prevention of the disease), and decline in productivity, through lost time. In the case of mortality, losses to households include lost future income and cumulative investment on the sick till death. Records of reported mortality from tropical diseases in Nigeria indicate that out of all major tropical diseases, malaria spells the greatest agony on households. Table 4.2 below shows that malaria is also a major source of mortality in Nigeria.

Table 4.2 Reported mortality from tropical diseases in Nigeria (period average)

Period	Filiaris	Onchocercariasis	Malaria	Schistosomiasis
1971-75	14	1	458	27
1976-80	2	4	1,439	10
1981-85	3	12	1,039	18
1986-90	6	9	1,675	20
1991-95	15	7	1,857	10

Source: Calculated from *FOS Statistical Bulletin* (Various Issues).

Reported mortality from malaria over the period shows that malaria was responsible for about ninety two per cent of total reported deaths from tropical diseases between 1971–1975; about ninety seven per cent between 1981–85 and well over ninety eight per cent within 1991–1995 (calculated from Table 4.2 above).

Inadequate data on malaria in the country to a very large extent limits attempt to exhaustively determine the connections between malaria incidence, mortality and poverty. Table 4.3 below relates the trend in reported malaria incidence to mortality and the level of poverty in Nigeria.

Table 4.3 Malaria morbidity, mortality and poverty in Nigeria

Year	Morbidity ('000)	Mortality	Poverty (%)
1980	1,171	865	28.1
1985	1,284	1,400	46.3
1992	1,219	1,337	42.7
1996	1,314	3,268	65.6

Source: FOS Statistical Bulletin (Various Issues) & FOS, 1999.

Although reported trends in incidence and mortality due to malaria are substantially lower than the actual trends, based on these figures, meaningful estimate on trend in malaria and poverty in Nigeria can be made. Table 4.3 indicates that the three variables moved in the same direction, though with different magnitudes, which may be an indication of existence of causality between malaria and poverty.

The connections between malaria and poverty come in a number of dynamic ways; at the household level, malaria affects the productivity of two major assets: people and their land. Households also frequently spend a substantial share of their income on malaria prevention and treatment, in addition to the effort they devote to the control of mosquito nuisance. The cost of prevention and treatment consumes scarce household resources. Households and individuals also spend a substantial part of their productive time caring for the ill, or seeking care.

In Sub-Saharan Africa (including Nigeria), households spend between $2 and $25 on malaria treatment and between $0.20 and $15 on prevention each month (Mills, 1998). As high as thirteen per cent of the total farm income in Nigeria is currently being used to treat malaria, but many households are simply too poor to be able to pay for adequate prevention and treatment of malaria (World Health Report, 1999). Each attack of malaria results in three – four days loss by each patient, with another three – four days of reduced productivity at work or school (WHO, 2001) apart from substantial time and resource loss by caregivers. The loss to households may however be greater with the current trend in malaria resistance to traditional first-line drugs (Mosanya, 1998). Such losses have serious implications for poor households who constitute over sixty five per cent of the nation's population (FOS, 1999) and live under pitiable conditions.

4.2 Literature Review

A substantial body of literature exists on the impact of health on the household economy and the gross domestic product (Baldwin and Weisbrod, 1974; Barlow, 1979; World Bank, 1993; Leighton *et al.,* 1993; Goodman *et al.,* 2000). Studies (Hamoudi and Sachs, 1999) indicate remarkable cross-country correlation between output per capita and some health indicators. Many of these studies suggest that health status is one of the most important determinants of economic success (Schultz, 1994; Nur, 1993; Sawyer, 1993). Gains from good health include opportunity to work maximally without being interrupted by illness, greater opportunities to obtain better paying jobs and longer working lives. These factors combine together to increase both the short and long term productivity of individuals, which is measured in the literature by earnings, including wages and salaries, and other remuneration other than transfers (Klarman, 1965).

The literature is specific on the economic impact of adult health (Bartel and Taubman, 1979; Hamoudi and Sachs, 1999; Over, 1992). The primary focus of most of these existing literatures has been the estimation of effects of ill-health on adult labor supply and earnings. However, a significant but well neglected issue in the literature on ill-health and poverty is the impact of an individual health status (especially children's health) on other members of the household (Pitt and Rosenzweig, 1990). Literature on the economic burden of malaria shows that quite a neglected area is the determination of burden of malaria on caregivers. Leighton *et al.,* (1993), a study on Kenya and Nigeria suggested that an important area of follow up on malaria in relation to productivity and poverty should include caregivers' behavior in relation to work and intra-household time allocation in the presence of malaria.

Although, many of the existing studies came up with notable results, in most cases, they failed to give sufficient attention to the complex effect of malaria burden on economic activities of household members. Researchers have found the effect of malaria on productivity insignificant in many instances, because adults who are regularly exposed to malaria tend to develop immunity, which subsequently shortens the period of malaria illness (Goodman *et al.*, 2000). Some adults endure malaria illness and partially participate in labor market activities and this reduces the economic loss due to malaria. Also, since affected children do not participate in market and non-market activities, apart from going to school, the effects of malaria illness in children are transferred to other household members. The actual impact of malaria in a high transmission area is manifested in the cost of caring for sick children and other vulnerable family members such as pregnant women (Goodman *et al.*, 2000).

With recent evidence on the status of malaria in Africa (MIM, 2001), an intensive focus on the burden of malaria on children and caregivers is pertinent. Focusing on such important issues as dynamic relationships between malaria in children, who are the most vulnerable groups (WHO, 1993), and the functioning of the household systems is quite important in the design of mechanisms for targeting poverty alleviation programs to needy groups. Initiating a target-oriented policy in malaria management programs is worthwhile, as malaria remains the deadliest public health problem in African countries today (Federal Ministry of Health, 1991; OAU, 1997). It is the biggest killer of children, a major "demobilizer" of labor productive capacity, and a cause of poverty (Federal Ministry of Health 1989; Hammer, 1993; Claessen *et al.*, 2001).

The costs of malaria include its burden on the individual, the household, and the whole economy. The economic burden of malaria can interestingly be studied from micro and macro-model viewpoints as in Castro and Mokate (1988). From the microeconomic point of view, malaria incidence directly affects performance, work hours, schooling, fertility, and physical health at birth, all of which affect current and future productivity.

From the macroeconomic viewpoint, malaria reduces growth potential of some industries, notably tourism, raises the cost of public health infrastructure. Some specific studies (Haworth, 1988; Gallup and Sachs, 1998; and Gallup, Sachs and Mellinger, 1998) after controlling for other factors, found that malaria exerts a significant adverse effect on economic growth. Also, McCarthy, Wolf and Wu (2000) found that countries with the highest level of malaria morbidity have not only the lowest initial growth rates of output per capita, but also that of human and physical capital.

4.3 Study Design and Data

This chapter focuses on the analysis of clinically confirmed malaria. It differs from various existing studies in this vein, which are often limited to self-reported cases of malaria. A hospital-based study is more accurate in estimating the total economic loss due to malaria. It enables us to determine quite well the costs associated with malaria, such as costs of consultation, medication, laboratory tests, and transportation to and from health facilities. Moreover, results from a hospital-based study are appropriate for making recommendations about how to improve procedures for treating malaria.

The survey for the chapter was carried out in Ibadan, Oyo State, a state known as an all year round malaria transmission zone. The two clinics in the state that are most frequently used by malaria patients, namely, the Adeoyo Hospital, and the University College Hospital (UCH), which are owned by the state and the federal authorities respectively, were surveyed. Both hospitals operate specialized malaria clinics. Adeoyo Hospital is located in the heart of a rural area (as defined by the National Population Commission) of Ibadan called Yemetu, while UCH is within the urban part of the city.

A multi-stage random sampling method was used to select the two clinics from other clinics. Stratified random sampling was used to select the caregivers who brought children with malaria to the hospital. The caregivers were interviewed once, and that was after the children had been screened for malaria in the wards and given treatment. The survey was carried out over a period of 8 weeks, with 500 cases being surveyed at each site, making a total of 1000 cases.

The survey focused on children aged one to sixty months since they constitute a group that is most vulnerable to malaria (WHO, 1996). The survey instrument had two sections; the first section requested information on the socio economic characteristics of the household members including the number of people living in a household, type of accommodation available, and environmental and living conditions. The second section of the questionnaire focused on the primary caregivers, whom comprised individuals that brought the sick children to the clinic.

The questionnaire was designed to get information on the total cost of treating a child afflicted with malaria. The questions focused on both the direct and the indirect cost of malaria. The cost of treating malaria include the direct cost as stated by mothers who are the primary caregivers, e.g. the cost of drugs, cost of round trip transportation to the health facility, duration of malaria bout, and whether or not school absenteeism occurred in the case of school going child. Included in the indirect cost is the opportunity cost of time spent caring for the sick child.

4.4 Cost Computation

4.4.1 Direct cost

Total direct cost of malaria includes all cash expenditure on malaria victims by the entire household, which comprises expenditure by the primary caregivers who accompany the sick child to the source of treatment. In computing direct cost, it was assumed that the transportation cost for the child to a source of treatment was free so that transport cost was computed for the number of individuals that accompanied the child multiplied by the number of times that they visited the hospital during the same malaria episode. The direct cost also includes the out-of-pocket expenditures for medicine before and after visiting the health facility.

4.4.2 Indirect cost

The indirect cost of illness includes the value of productive time lost and income forgone not only by malaria patients but also by the caregivers. In the case of the labor hired to replace the caregivers, the amount paid to such labor is part of the indirect cost of a malaria episode. The opportunity cost of the time the caregivers allocate to illness is a good measure of indirect burden of malaria (Becker, 1965). However, since households allocate their time between market and leisure activities, there is controversy as to which of the time element (labor or leisure) is actually lost in the event of illness. We tried to overcome this controversy by assuming that in most cases, visitation to a health facility coincides with periods of labor shortages within a household.

The lost workdays were valued at a local daily wage rate, which was applied according to categories of caregivers. An assumption made in applying this rate is that children do not perform market work. However, children's school work that was lost due to malaria was valued at wages prevailing in local labor markets. The lost days as a result of malaria, which is a theoretical reflection of lost income, depends on the nature of work and terms of employment. For instance, workers with paid sick leave or with monthly salaries do not lose income when they miss work due to care giving as the self-employed persons do. It was assumed that all civil-service employees enjoy sick leave benefit and therefore do not lose income during episodes of malaria in a household.

Valuation of the cost of time spent on a malaria illness involves the following: an assessment of the number of workdays the caregiver lost in order to take care of the sick child; the time spent at the health facility waiting for or going through consultations and laboratory tests; and the time spent traveling to and from the health facility.

There is need to convert the time cost of illness as indicated above, into a monetary value. The average daily wage rate (a theoretical measure of labor productivity) was used to value the amount of time lost due to malaria to obtain an estimate of an indirect cost of a case of malaria or fever.

4.5 Findings

Fever, as defined by the medical reporting system in Sub-Saharan Africa, has been found to closely correspond to the clinical diagnosis of malaria (Shepard *et al.*, 1991). This is confirmed in this study as respondents often use fever and malaria interchangeably.

The study confirms the general finding in the literature that the bulk of malaria patients are children. It further shows that the economic loss due to childhood malaria is greater than the malaria burden associated with the other population groups put together. Treatment of malaria in children is costlier, because severely ill children usually need intensive care. The direct cost of childhood malaria is small relative to the opportunity cost of the time spent to care for ill children. The study disaggregates children caretakers into three groups, namely: formal employees, self-employed and unemployed persons.

4.5.1 Characteristics of caregivers

About ninety per cent of the caregivers of sick children are biological mothers. Disaggregating the caregivers sample by occupation or activity shows that 910 of the caregivers were self-employed, sixty of them were government employees and thirty were unemployed. The mean working hours for the total sample was about 8.69 hours per day. This mean varies by activity type as follows: nine hours for self-employed persons, eight hours for government employees and nine hours for unemployed caregivers.

According to the survey, the mean daily income for all individuals in the sample is ₦712.81. Disaggregating the mean daily earnings by employment status, the self-employed persons earn an average of ₦725.76 per day and government employees collect ₦750.24 daily. We value the daily domestic activities often affected by sickness in the case of unemployed persons using the hourly wage rate prevailing in the local labor market. The minimum pay in the local labor market was an average of ₦325.00 per day. On the average the total household monthly income was ₦43,040.22. Disaggregating the total household income with respect to caregivers employment status we have ₦45,039.64 for self-employed, ₦20,758.00 for government employees and ₦26,955.68 for unemployed family members.

The survey further reveals that ninety eight per cent of the primary caregivers were married and seventy two per cent of them were of Islamic religion. Only forty per cent of the surveyed individuals were literate. The remaining sixty per cent were without any formal schooling. The majority of the households with children who had malaria symptoms were large, with five persons or more. The average age of the sick child seen at the clinic was twenty seven months; and in nearly every case, malaria was the reason for the visit.

4.5.2 Prevalence of malaria

In the clinic samples, malaria was reported as the major illness in children. The survey shows that 72.2 per cent of the primary caregivers indicated that malaria was the main cause of morbidity in children. About twenty five per cent of caregivers reported that diarrhea was a common health problem in children, another 1.6 per cent identified breathing problem, while about one per cent acknowledged incidence of cold. These responses correspond to Ekanem's (1991) findings on the five most common health problems in children in Nigeria (figure 4.1 and table 4.1; also see appendix tables 4.A1–4.A6).

Figure 4.1 Major health problems in children in Nigeria.

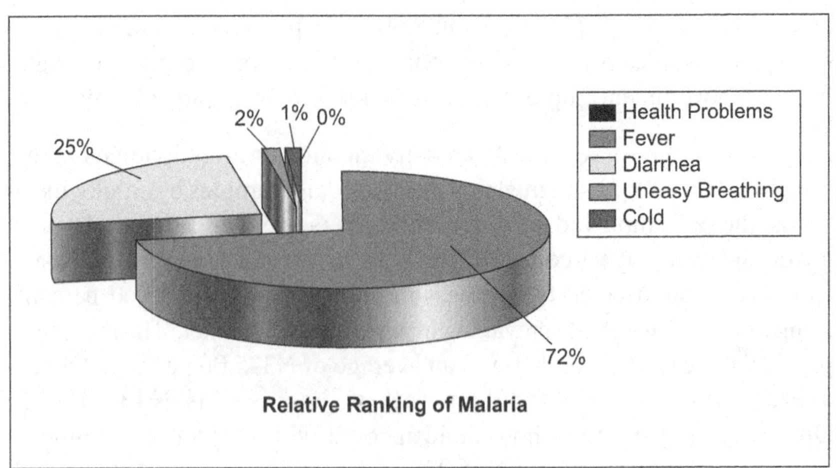

4.5.3 Beliefs about malaria

The respondents associated malaria in children with the following signs: temperature, loss of appetite and activity, vomiting and uneasy breathing, headaches and diarrhea. Disaggregating the caretakers by literacy status, similar pattern was found in beliefs about malaria in both literate and illiterate individuals (figure 4.2 and table 4.2).

From figure 4.2, it can be seen that thirty eight per cent and 40.3 per cent of illiterate and literate caregivers respectively identified abnormal increase in temperature as the major sign of malaria in children. Vomiting or cold was also significantly reported by the two groups. For instance, the figure shows that as much as 37.6 per cent and 26.8 per cent of literate and illiterate samples respectively identified vomiting and cold with malaria. The same proportion of illiterate sample associated loss of appetite and uneasy breathing with malaria in children compared with 16.8 per cent and 5.3 per cent among literate individuals.

The caregivers beliefs about causes of malaria or fever show a similar pattern. Mosquito's infective bite is recognized by about the same proportion of literate and illiterate population as the most frequent cause of malaria in children. About eighty nine per cent of literate and eighty nine per cent of illiterate caregivers in this sample believe that mosquito bite is the medium

Figure 4.2 Identified symptoms of malaria in children by caretaker's education

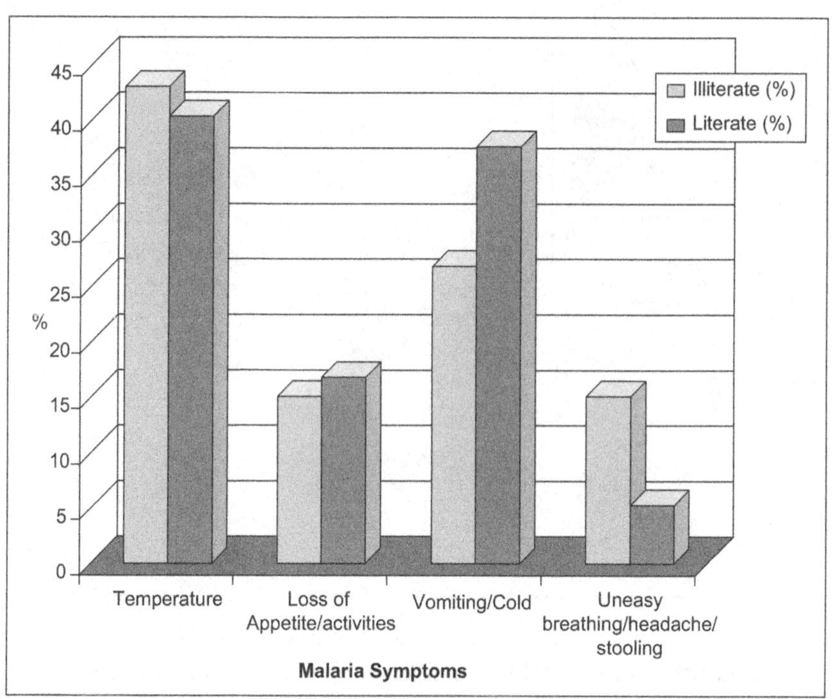

of malaria transmission. About seven per cent and four per cent of literate caregivers identified heat and teething as the respective causes of malaria in children compared with five per cent among illiterate persons.

4.5.4 Management of malaria

The caregivers first treated malaria at home, usually with western medicine, before taking further action.

Figure 4.3 shows that ninety two per cent of the sample gave anti-malarial drugs to children at home on perceiving the symptoms associated with malaria. During an episode of malaria, the caregivers bought drugs from local drug retailers and in many instances used drugs that were left over after treatment of a previous malaria illness. Only seven per cent of the caretakers initially sought help from a health facility after noticing a malaria symptom in children.

Figure 4.3 Management of malaria by place of treatment (%)

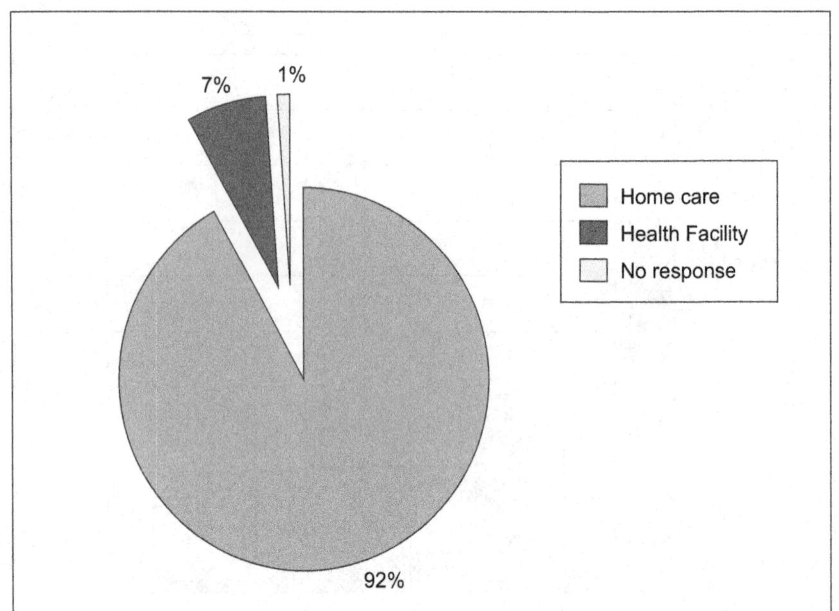

The data further shows that the elapsed time before a child was taken to a clinic on recognition of malaria symptom ranged from one to thirty days. None of the caregivers took a sick child to the clinic within the first two days of the illness. It seems that parents consider clinical action necessary only when they have exhausted possibilities of home remedies. Figure 4.4 shows the amount of time elapsed before a visit to a clinic by occupation category of caregivers.

Figure 4.4 reveals that caregivers in Nigeria underestimate the seriousness of malaria because over half of the total sample took the sick children to the clinic after three to five days upon recognizing the onset of the disease. Across all occupational categories, visits to clinics were made at least two days after recognition of malaria. The majority of the caregivers resorted to care seeking in the clinics within the third and fifth days after the onset of malaria (figure 4.4).

About sixty per cent of unemployed caregivers opted for clinical treatment within the first three – five days of illness recognition compared with 47.4

per cent and 46.7 per cent among the self-employed and the civil servants. Note that over forty six per cent of civil servants opted for clinical care after the fifth day. About 13.3 per cent neglected taking clinical actions until after fifteen days had elapsed since the onset of the illness. The high percentage of unemployed caregivers seeking clinical treatment for malaria relatively earlier may be due to the fact that they have more time to spare, unlike the self-employed and the government employed. Initial significant neglect of clinical care by the government employees may be explained by the difficulties encountered in re-allocation of time from paid job to care-giving.

Figure 4.4 Time to clinical action taken after the onset of illness by occupation of caregivers

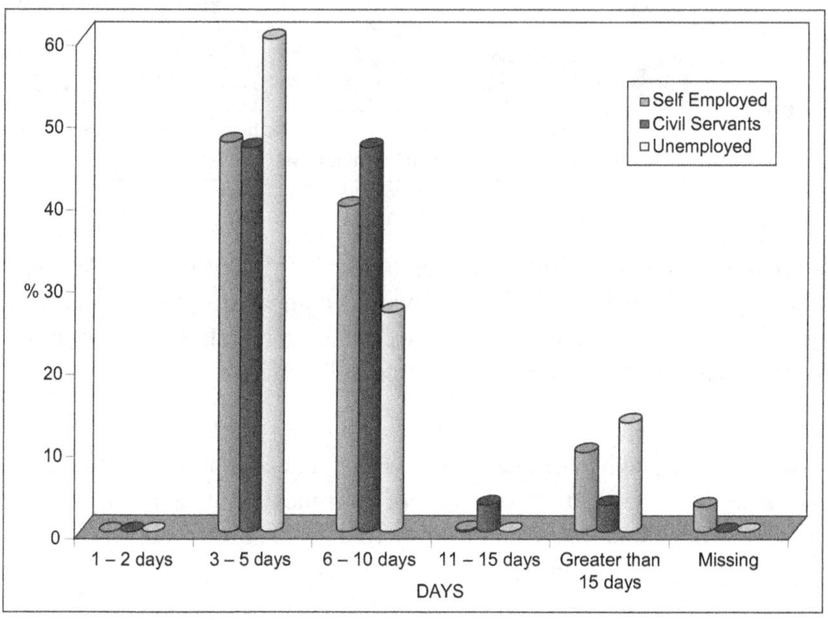

4.5.5 Malaria prevention

A large number of caregivers (50%) reported practicing at least one form of malaria prevention. The majority of respondents used nets on doors or windows as a way of preventing malaria transmission. One interesting observation here is the minor role of education in respect of the prevention

Figure 4.5 Malaria preventive measures by caretaker' literacy (%)

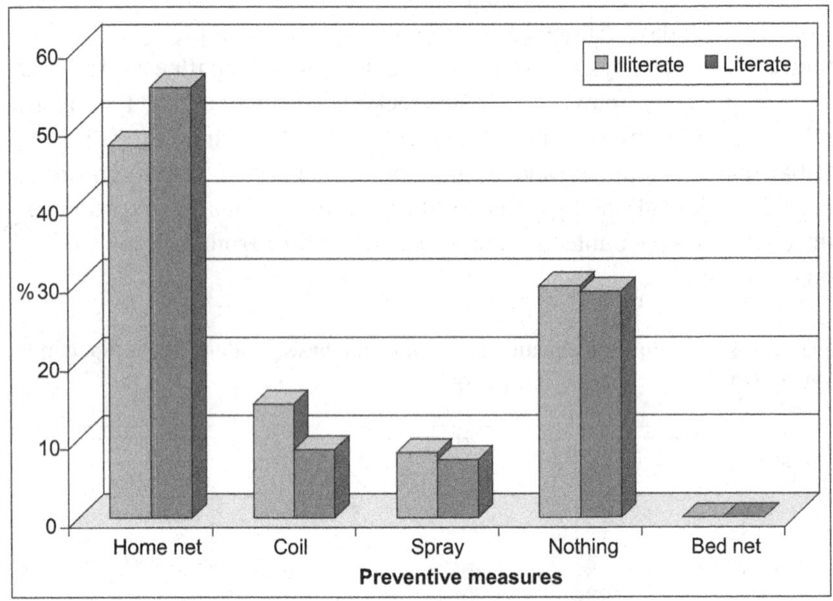

activities undertaken. The literate individuals (55% of the sample) used home-nets to prevent malaria transmission compared with fifty per cent among illiterate persons. As to the use of coil and insecticide sprays, more illiterates use coils and sprays compared to literate persons (figure 4.5).

It is surprising that none of the caregivers in the sample has ever-used an insecticide treated bed net, despite its effectiveness in preventing malaria. The main explanation for this is lack of awareness of the existence of this prevention method. More than twenty five per cent of caregivers did not use any prevention method.

4.5.6 Cost of childhood malaria

Direct cost

The direct cost of malaria includes expenditure on drugs, round-trip transportation expenses to and from health facilities, and expenditure on prevention activities undertaken at home. Generally, the total direct cost of malaria includes out-of-pocket expenses on treatments plus subsidies provided by the state government for malaria management and control. However, the area of focus in this study was total private expenditure on malaria treatment and prevention.

For more than ninety per cent of the sick children, the first line anti-malaria drugs were recommended by health care providers. The survey reveals that the average direct cost of a bout of malaria in a child among the unemployed caregivers ranked the highest at ₦686.87, followed by the cost among the self-employed caregivers, which averaged at ₦490.17 and was lowest for the government employed caregivers at ₦ 478.49 (Table 4.4).

The magnitude of the average direct cost of malaria across different categories of caregivers is correlated with financial commitments to malaria prevention activities. It can be seen from table 4.4 that the unemployed spent the least on prevention activities, and this probably accounts for the higher malaria burden in they bear.

Table 4.4 Direct costs of treating a case of fever in children by employment status of primary care giver (sample size = 1000)

Cost Category	Self-Employed		Government Employed		Unemployed		Total Average
	₦	$US	₦	$US	₦	$US	₦
Treatment	420.06	3.82	379.11	3.45	509.09	4.63	420.27
Transportation	70.11	0.64	99.38	0.90	177.78	1.62	75.09
Cost per Episode	490.17	4.46	478.49	4.35	686.87	6.24	495.76
Cost of Preventive Measures	146.42	1.33	206.00	1.87	120.00	1.09	149.30

Source: Survey, 2001.

Intra-household distribution of malaria burden

Expenditure on malaria was classified into financial expenses on drugs and medical consultations and the expense on transportation to and from health facilities. The survey reveals that the bulk of cost of treating children was

Table 4.5 Intra-household distribution of expenses on malaria in children

Employment Status of Caregiver	Status of Caregiver Within a Household (N =1000)			
	Cost of Medical Treatment (₦)		Other Cost (₦)	
	Father or Husband	Mothers or Wife	Father or Husband	Mother or Wife
Self-employed	420.06	0.0	0.0	70.11
Government employed	379.11	0.0	0.0	99.38
Unemployed	509.09	0.0	177.78	0.0

Source: Survey data.

borne by husbands (Table 4.5). This finding might be a reflection of the role husbands play in the control and allocation of family resources.

Irrespective of the employment status of household heads and their spouses, the expenditure on malaria treatment was largely borne by husbands or fathers. However, other costs such as transport and associated expenses were borne by mothers except in the case of unemployed caregivers where fathers or husbands bore the entire financial burden of treating children. In the case of the self-employed caregivers, fathers bore as much as 79.2 per

Table 4.6 Time spent on malaria episode on treatment related activities by employment status of a caregiver (N =1000)

Time Category	Self-Employed	Government Employed	Unemployed	Total
Traveling Time (bus)	15 minutes	23 minutes	45 minutes	17 minutes
Waiting Time	3 hours	3 hours	3 hours	3 hours
Time with the Doctor	45 minutes	25 minutes	40 minutes	44 minutes
Time on Laboratory Tests	4 hours	4 hours	4 hours	4 hours
Time in Dispensary	30 minutes	30 minutes	30 minutes	30 minutes
Total	**8hrs 30min**	**8hrs 18min**	**8hrs 50min**	**9hrs 43min**

Source: Survey data.

cent of the total financial expense. The indirect cost consisted of the productive time lost by the sick persons as well as the caregivers. Productive time loss includes school days lost or time spent seeking care (Table 4.6).

4.5.7 Time lost by the sick and caregivers

On average each bout of malaria lasted about six days. Both the sick and caregivers lost the same number of productive days. The days lost to malaria by the sick and the caregivers differed by age of the sick child. For school age children, their loss was the number of school days missed, while for children under school going age, the loss was limited to days of inactivity or the number of days they could not play.

The average number of complete days lost to clinically confirmed malaria averaged six days per episode. The actual average productive time lost to a single episode was about fifty three hours for the whole sample. In the disaggregated sample, the government employed lost fewer days and hours, with the loss of thirty six hours, which consisted of complete two working days of 16 working hours and incomplete four days of twenty hours. Both self employed and unemployed persons lost six full working days, i.e., fifty four hours and sixty hours respectively per episode. Average traveling time for the total sample is seventeen minutes, with unemployed persons spending an average of forty five minutes in transit to health facilities; government employed spent on average twenty three minutes; and self employed spent an average of fifteen minutes.

Table 4.7 Time spent on non-treatment related activities per malaria episode by employment status of a caregiver (N =1000)

Time category	Self-Employed	Government Employed	Unemployed	Total Sample
Incomplete Days on Care of the Sick	–	4 days 20 hours	6 days 60hrs	6 days 53hrs 1min
Complete Days on Care of the Sick	6 54hrs	2 16hrs	–	–
Total Time	54hrs	36hrs	60hrs	53hrs 1min
Estimated Cost of Time Lost Per Episode	₦4,354.56	₦3,376.08	₦2,166.60	₦4,348.96

Source: Survey data.

Across the entire sample, an average of three hours was lost waiting to consult doctors, while an additional average of forty four minutes was spent with doctors. For the laboratory test to confirm the presence of malaria or otherwise, on average four hours were required. The alternatives available to conduct laboratory tests were private clinics that charged between ₦250 and ₦300 per single round of laboratory test. Drug dispensing took an average of thirty minutes in all facilities.

On average, all caregivers lost a total of fifty three hours per bout of malaria, which amounted to ₦4348.96 for the entire sample. Estimated indirect cost per episode of malaria by employment status was as follows: ₦4354.56 in the case of the self-employed, ₦3376.08 in the case of government employees and ₦2166.60 among the unemployed. Pertinent to the above cost figures is the following information:

(a) The number of days is multiplied by the average number of hours spent in income generating activity and household chores. An average of nine and eight hours are spent on income generating activities by self-employed and government employed respectively while an average of nine hours is reported by the unemployed caregivers on household chores.

(b) Incomplete days imply that only five hours of productive service put into government job per day, the rest of the day is taken off in order to take care of the sick child.

(c) In the case of the unemployed, minimum wage income of hired substitutes per day is ₦325; thus an hourly income of ₦36.11 is used as the conversion factor.

For the self-employed and the government employed reported average incomes of ₦725.76 and ₦750.24 per day, which means an hourly income of ₦80.64, 93.78 respectively were used. The hourly incomes were deflated by those hours used in productive venture for each of the groups.

From the study, 100 per cent of the sick children of school age do not go to school during the period of malaria attacks. The ailment has the greatest implication for the self-employed mothers who leave everything in order to take care of sick children. This means for complete six days, neither the

Table 4.8 Total expenditure per episode of fever in a child (N = 1000)

Cost item	Self-employed	Exp as % of hh Income	Govt. Emp-loyed	Exp as % of hh Income	Unemp-loyed	Exp as % of hh Income	Total Sample	Exp as % of hh Income
Direct Cost	₦490.17	1.09	₦478.49	2.31	₦686.87	2.55	₦495.36	1.15
Indirect cost	₦4354.56	9.67	₦3376.08	16.26	₦2166.60	8.04	₦4348.96	10.10
Total Cost	₦4844.73	10.76	₦3854.57	18.57	₦2853.47	10.59	₦4844.32	11.26
Total Cost (US$)	44.04		35.04		25.94		39.54	

Source: Survey data.

self-employed mother nor the sick child does any productive venture. Also, the unemployed mothers lose as many days as the self-employed. The difference, however, is that the opportunity cost of the unemployed time is far lesser than the former. In the case of the government employed, an average of two days is completely dedicated to the sick child. While the four other days are incomplete working days, that is, they leave the office by twelve before the close of day's job not to go back for the rest of the day. This shows that in the case of government employees, the state bears the loss associated with malaria management, mainly because irrespective of absenteeism, the government still goes ahead to pay their salaries for the unproductive period.

Figure 4.6 Components per episode of fever in a child (%)

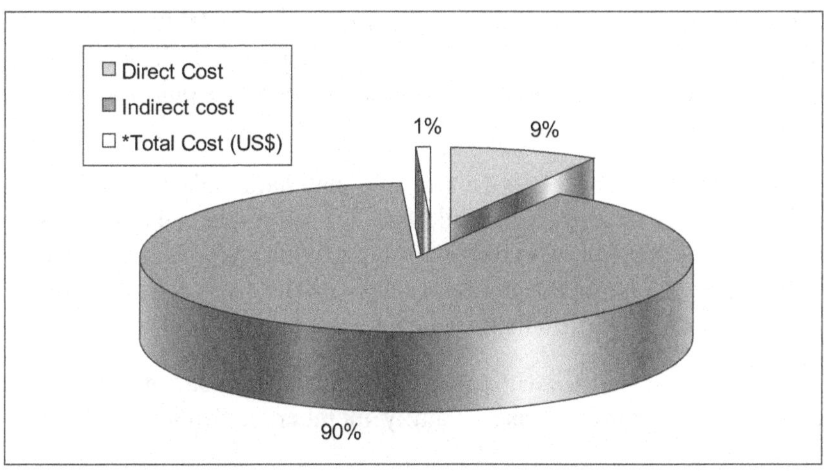

4.5.8 Total cost of a single bout of malaria

Table 4.8 gives the summary of the total cost of a single bout of malaria per child using the actual expenditure by caregivers and their spouses, and the monetized indirect cost of care-seeking. Converting the total cost by a rate of about ₦110.00 = US$1.00, we have average cost for the total sample as US$39.54. For the disaggregated sample, average cost per episode of malaria is US$44.04 for self-employed, US$35.04 for government employed, and the average cost of unemployed caregiver is US$19.70.

Table 4.8 gives the total expenditure on a single bout of malaria in children as a percentage of the households' monthly income. The last column of the table shows that the average expenditure per bout of malaria in a child within the household is well over ten per cent of the individual household's income.

4.6 Discussion and Conclusions

The study reveals that so much of human, financial and material resources are constantly being lost to malaria incidence in Nigeria. For a typical African society with usually large families, implication of malaria attack on family members is likely to be more damaging to the household's income and income earning potential, consumption, family savings and investment. For households already living below the poverty line, uncontrolled malaria attack may keep them permanently in poverty, and the currently growing trend of malaria incidence is also capable of creating a new class of the poor. It is also recognized that beyond the clinical time lost by primary caregivers, the actual number of hours wasted on avoidable incidence of malaria is more, as more of the household members contribute their own quota to care giving, opportunity cost of which is not accounted for in this study.

Majority of our respondents believe that malaria is indeed a major and most notorious of diseases in children. The caregivers who are mostly mothers have peculiar ways of identifying malaria probably based on past experiences and familiar signs associated with the disease, and in most of the cases doctors confirm their suspicion.

The signs often identified with malaria can be a starting point of household's education about the disease. Family members and malaria endemic communities deserve to be given greater awareness on the dynamics of the disease, particularly with the current increasing incidence of severe and drug resistant malaria. Some households and communities may require new orientation using their basic knowledge and beliefs, and the formula for identifying the disease as a basic ingredient for massive community-wide education in the prevention and control of the disease.

The survey indicates that mothers are usually the primary agents in managing malaria cases at the household level. In over ninety per cent of malaria cases, mothers bear major non-financial responsibilities for managing the sick. The data also reveals that over ninety per cent of the cases are first and foremost managed at home. This implies that the most important sets of decisions such as the management system to adopt, the kind of drugs to use and the status of the disease are taken by the mothers, as the primary caregivers. Home care for malaria patient is the first and mostly favored approach by caregivers, while decision to go to the proximate health facility is mostly taken when cases deteriorate. Determinants of malaria management systems (whether to use home care or the health facility) include accessibility, promptness of care, cost (both travel and treatment) and effectiveness of treatment. The analysis shows that:

- There is need for non-formal and even formal training of mothers who are usually the primary caregivers so as to be able to determine the characteristics and proper management strategies for the disease.
- Most mothers who are the primary caregivers are reportedly put off by time wastage at health facilities. More specialized equipments (for instance laboratory equipment) are required to enable prompt diagnostic tests as well as general improvement in service rendered.
- Stakeholders should initiate continuous training on identification of complicated malaria; proper management of uncomplicated malaria cases by making certified and specially pre-packaged drugs available; enforcement of counter counseling on appropriate medication and dosage; proper storage of essential drugs and hazards associated with the use of self-medications.

For almost all caregivers, it took a while before taking the decision to attend clinics; the data shows that none of the cases were reported in the hospital until the third day of the illness. Self-determined care at home however, encourages delicate management lapses, including the use of wrong drugs and wrong dosage. In a number of cases, drug administrations are suspended as soon as the patient improves and the remaining drugs kept for future use. Home medication is also often characterized by untimely administration and improper counseling, and probable complication of supposedly uncomplicated cases.

The implication of the above for severity of malaria and current trend in malaria resistance to essential drugs is serious. Mothers should be encouraged to seek professional care in clinics as early as possible and be made aware of the deadly implications of incomplete drug dosage and improper management of cases. Access to home-test kit is essential and should be made available and affordable.

In the case of treated bed nets, it is surprising that despite the hues and cries about the effectiveness of ITN, 100 per cent of the respondents were not aware of where this important preventive measure is available. Many people are not aware of any established distribution system or center. It is recommended that:

- Bed nets should be made available in all health facilities and other accessible areas;
- Awareness campaigns should be initiated so that the populace may be acquainted with the importance of this preventive measure;
- Subsidies on essential antimalaria facilities should be encouraged;
- Private sector should be encouraged to produce and distribute insecticides-treated bed nets.

The study confirms that the negative impact of malaria on households and national economy is indeed increasing. The focus group discussion by Leighton *et al* (1993) on Nigeria suggests three complete days lost per round of malaria incidence. Our study however recorded an average of four to six days of complete incapacitation depending on the employment status of the primary caregivers. Malaria is claiming more days, more resources and creating new sets of the poor in Nigeria. With the deteriorating level of per capita income and substantial resources being lost per bout of malaria, combined with average increasing number of bouts per year, we can be sure of deepening poverty within the household system which trickles down to worsening national poverty.

This study also reveals that the third party effect of malaria far exceeds the direct impact on the sick, and that mothers bear the greatest burden of caregiving despite significant financial burden borne by the fathers or husbands. The current trend in the disease among children and increasing economic loss deserves renewed attention. Target oriented approach to poverty alleviation should have consideration for children and women. Well-focused malaria management policies that have a gender sensitive approach to poverty alleviation often identify women as more effective managers of household resources; and yet most resource allocation decisions are in the hands of men, a situation that needs to change.

The relationship between commitment to prevention and level of malaria incidence, and the associated expenditure by employment status of care givers suggests that increased commitment is a necessity in reducing the overall burden of malaria in Nigeria. Greater commitment to preventive measures will no doubt reduce the physical, financial and time resources burden on the households. This may trickle down to increased consumption, savings and investment by the households. The implication of this is the greater propensity for the households to stay off the poverty line, while there is greater likelihood for both the household and national welfare to be substantially enhanced depending on the access to and state of the labor market.

References

Baldwin, R.E. and Weisbrod, B.A. (1974), "Disease and Labor Productivity". *Economic Development and Cultural Change* 22: 414–35.

Barlow, R. (1979), "Health and Economics Development : A Theoretical and Empirical Review". *Research in Human Capital and Development* 1: 45–75.

Bartel, A. and Taubman, P. (1979), "Health and Labor Market Success: The Role of Various Diseases". *Review of Economics and Statistics* 61 (1): 1–8

Becker, G. (1965), "A Theory of the Allocation of Time". *Economic Journal,* September.

Claeson, M. *et al.,* (2001), "Health, Nutrition and Population", Mimeo.

Castro, E.B. and Mokate, K.M. (1988), "Malaria and its Socio-Economic Meanings: The Study of Cunlay in Columbia, in Alandro N.H and Patricia Rossenfield (ed.), *Economics, Health and Tropical Disease.* Manila: University of Phillipines.

Denison, E.F. (1967), "The Sources of Economic Growth in the USA and the Alternatives Before us". *Supplementary Paper* No.13. New York: Committee for Economic Development.

Ekanem, O.J. (1997), Keynote Address – Malaria in Nigeria: Two-Day National Symposium on Malaria in Nigeria, 4–5 November.

Ejezie, G.C., Ezedinachi, E.N.U., Usanga, E.A. , Gemande, E.I., Ikpatt, N.W., and Alaribe, A.A. (1990), "Malaria and its Treatment in Villages of Aboh Mbaise, Imo State, Nigeria". *Acta Tropica* 48 (1).

Federal Ministry of Health (1991), *Bamako Initiative Management Manual.* Lagos: Nigeria, FMH.

Fogel, R.W. (1991), "New Sources and New Techniques for the Study of Secular Trends in Nutritional Status, Health Mortality and the Process of Ageing", NBER Working Paper, 26, Cambridge MA (May).

Gallup, J. L. and Sachs, J.D. (2001), "The Economic Burden of Malaria". *The American Journal of Topical Medicine and Hygiene* 64 (Suppl. 1).

Gallup, J. L. and Sachs, J.D. (2000), "The Economic Burden of Malaria", Centre for International Development, Working Paper No 52 (July), Harvard University.

_______ (1998), "Geography and Economic Development", *Brookings Paper of Economic Activity.*

_______ and Mellinger (1998), "Geography and Economic Development", Annual World Bank Conference on Development. Washington D.C: World Bank.

Goodman, C., Coleman, P. and Mills, A. (2000), *Economic Analysis of Malaria Control in Sub Saharan Africa*. Switzerland: Global Forum for Health Research.

Hammer, J. (1993), "The Economics of Malaria Control". *World Bank Research Observer* 8 (1): 1–22.

Hamoudi, A.A. and Sachs, J.D. (1999), "Economic Consequences of Health Status: A Review of Evidence", CID Working Paper No. 30, Harvard University, Mimeo.

Haworth, J. (1988), "The Global Distribution of Malaria and Present Control Effort", in: Walter and McGregor (ed.), *Malaria: Principle and Practice of Malariology.* Edinburgh: Churchill Livingstone.

Klarman, H. (1965), "Socio-economic Impact of Heart Diseases", paper presented at the Heart Circulation Second National Conference on Cardiovascular Diseases. Washington, D.C.: US Government Printing Office.

Leighton, C., Foster, R. (1993), *Economic Impact of Malaria in Kenya and Nigeria*, Bethesda. Maryland: Abt Associates.

McCarthy, F.D,. *et al.*, (2000), "Malaria and Growth", A World Bank Working Paper on Health and Population, Nutrition, Fertility and HIV/AIDS. Washington D.C: The World Bank.

Mills, A. (1998), "Operational Research on the Economics of Insecticide-Treated Mosquito Nets: Lessons of Experience". *Annal of Tropical Medicine and Parasitology* 92 (4).

Mosanya, M.E. (1997), "National Malaria Policy–Plan of Action", Abstracts of a Two-Day National Symposium on Malaria in Nigeria.

Multilateral Initiative of Malaria (2001), "The Intolerable Burden of Malaria: A New Look at Numbers". *The American Journal of Tropical Medicine and Hygiene* (forthcoming).

Mwabu, G. (2001), "Poverty and Malaria in Africa: Research and Policy Agenda", Background Paper Prepared for Poverty and Malaria in Africa, AERC, Nairobi, Kenya.

Nur, E.T.M. (1993), "The Impact of Malaria on Labor Use and Efficiency in Sudan". *Social Science and Medicine.*

Nur, E.T.M. and Mahnam, H. (1986), "The Effects of Health on Agricultural Labor Supply: A Theoretical and Empirical Investigation", in: A. Herrin and Patricia Rosenfield, (eds.) *Economics, Health and Tropical Disease*. Manila University of Phillipines.

Organization of African Unity (1997), "Harare Declaration on Malaria Prevention and Control in the Context of African Economic Recovery and Development", Assembly of Heads of State and Government, June.

Over, M. (1992), *The Macroeconomic Impact of AIDS in Sub-Saharan Africa*, Population and Human Resources Department, World Bank.

Pitt, M. and Rosenzweig, M.R. (1990), "Estimating Intra-Household Incidence of Illness: Child Health and Gender Inequality in the Allocation of Time". *International Economic Review* 31 (4).

Roll Back Malaria, "The Abuja Declaration, Part 3", April 25, 2000. Abuja, Nigeria.

Sawyer, D. (1993), "Economic and Social Consequences of Malaria in New Colonization Projects in Brazil". *Social Science and Medicine* 37 (9).

Schultz, T.P. and Tansel, A. (1993), "Measurement of Returns to Adult Health: Morbidity Effects on Wage Rate in Cote d'Ivoire and Ghana", *LSMS Working Paper* No. 95. The World Bank, (April).

Schultz, T. P. (1994), "Human Capital, Family Planning and their Effect on Population Growth". *American Economic Review* 84 (2).

_______ (1961) "Investment in Human Capital". *The American Economic Review* 51(1).

Sevilla-Casas, E. (1993), "Human Mobility and Malaria risk in the Naya River of Colombia". *Social Science and Medicine* 37 (9).

Shepard, D.S., Ettling, M.B., Brinkman, U., and Saverborn, R. (1991), "The Economic Cost of Malaria in Africa". *Tropical Medicine and Parasitology* 42 (3).

Strauss, J. and Thomas, D. (1995), "Human Resources: Empirical Modelling of Household and Family Decisions", in: J .Behrman and T.N. Srinivasan, (eds.) *Handbook of Development Economics*, Vol. III.

Weller, T.H. (1958), "Tropical Medicine", in: *Encyclopedia Britannica*. Chicago: William Bennett.

Weisbrod, B.A. (1961), *Economics of Public Health: Measuring the Economic Impact of Diseases*. Philadelphia: University of Pennsylvania Press.

World Bank (1980), *Poverty and Human Development*. Washington D.C: The World Bank.

_______ (1993), *Investing in Health: World Development Report*. New York: Oxford University Press.

World Health Organization (1996), *WHO, 58–64, Technical Report Series, No. 735*. World Health Organization Expert Committee on Malaria, 18th report.

World Health Organization (2000), *Malaria Desk Situation Analysis – Nigeria*.

World Health Organization (2000), "Severe and Complicated Malaria". *Trans R. Soc. Trop. Med. Hyg.* 94 (suppl).

World Health Organization (1999), *World Health Report: Making a Difference*. Geneva Switzerland: World Health Organization.

Chapter 4 Appendix Tables

Table 4.A1 Ranking of major health problems in children

Health Problems	Ranking by Population in % (N = 1010)
Fever	72.2
Diarrhea	25.2
Uneasy Breathing	1.6
Cold	1.0

Source: Survey data.

Table 4.A2 Identified symptoms of malaria in children by caretakers' education (N = 1000)

Symptom	Illiterate (%)	Literate (%)	Total Population (%)
Temperature	43	40.3	52.
Loss of Appetite/ Activities	15.1	16.8	15.5
Vomiting/Cold	26.8	37.6	29.9
Uneasy Breathing/ Headache/ Stooling	15.1	5.3	2.6

Source: Survey 2001.

Table 4.A3 Beliefs about the causes of malaria by caregivers' literacy (N = 1000)

Belief	Literate	Illiterate	Total
Mosquito	89.1	89.2	89.2
Heat	6.9	5.4	6.4
Teething	4.0	5.4	4.4

Source: Survey data.

Table 4.A4 Type of action taken after the onset of illness (N = 1000)

Type of Action	% of Caretakers
Home Care	92.0
Health Facility	7.0
No Response	1.0

Source: Survey data.

Table 4.A5 Time to clinical action after the onset of illness by occupation of caregivers (N = 1000)

Time Clinical Action was Taken After Onset of Illness (days)	Self Employed	Civil Servants	Unemployed	Total
1 – 2 days	0	0	0	0
3 – 5 days	47.4	46.7	60.0	48.6
6 – 10 days	39.6	46.7	26.7	39.6
11 – 15 days	0.2	3.3	0	0.4
Greater Than 15 days	9.7	3.3	13.3	9.4
Missing	3.1	0	0	2.0

Source: Survey data.

Table 4.A6 Preventive measures by caretakers' literacy (N = 1000)

Preventive Measure	Illiterate (%)	Literate (%)	Total
Home Net	47.6	55.0	49.8
Coil	14.5	8.7	12.8
Spray	8.3	7.4	8.0
Nothing	29.6	28.9	29.4
Bed Net	0	0	0

Source: Survey data.

Chapter 5

The Demand for Malaria Control Products and Services: Evidence from Yaounde, Cameroon

Bernadette Dia Kamgnia

5.0 Introduction

In many developing countries, particularly in Sub-Saharan Africa, malaria has for several decades, remained one of the major public health problems. In Cameroon, malaria is still a serious problem by any measure. Studies show that it is the first cause of morbidity and of mortality for the entire population (MSP, 1998). In the work sector, it is believed to be the major reason for absenteeism; and in healthcare centers, a large majority of consultations are malaria related. Indeed, since 1985, Plasmodium falciparum, the major malaria vector, has become nationwide resistant to chloroquine, a medicine which is considered to be the principal treatment base for malaria (Louis, *et al.,* 1994).

To deal with such a preoccupying situation, anti-vectorial practices have been developed with emphasis on the use of chemical products (sprays and serpentines). Unfortunately, the cost of these practices is rather high, and constitutes a major financial burden for the households (Goff *et al.,* 1994). The tendency nowadays is for the vulgarization of the use of insecticide-treated bed nets.

This chapter analyzes the determinants of the demand for malaria control products and services in the specific case of the urban community of Yaoundé. Given that the effectiveness of a control approach requires first of all, the knowledge of the target populations' attitudes and practices with respect to malaria and the insecticide-treated bed nets, it is necessary to start by assessing the behavior of the households. Such analysis would shed light on the interventions most suited to the specificities of the aforesaid populations. The second section presents the objectives and hypotheses of the study, while the third section develops the study methodology. The major results of the study are discussed in the fourth section, while the fifth section concludes.

5.1 The Scope of Malaria in Cameroon

Cameroon is a Central African country that stretches over a 475,650-km² area. Located between the 2nd and 13th degrees of the northern latitude and the 9th and 16th degrees of the eastern longitude, it has a diversified tropical climate. The hot and wet seasons of this climate are particularly favorable to the development of tropical diseases like malaria and the onchocerciasis. From an administrative standpoint, the country is divided into ten provinces, fifty eight departments and 269 districts. On the medical standpoint, the organization of the health sector replicates that of the African scenario of medical system in three bodies: The central body, is composed of the ministry of public health, five directorates and two divisions, which deal with the general policy and, the design and implementation of the strategies. The intermediate unit, made up of the ten provincial divisions of the Ministry of Public Health, and the affiliated technical services, provides technical assistance to the districts in the implementation of health programs. Finally, the peripheral units, made up of 144 district health centers and the integrated health centers, implement the various health programs and activities.

5.1.1 The socioeconomic and medical profile of Cameroon

The demographic profile of Cameroon is characterized by an average annual growth rate of 2.9 per cent. In 2000, the population was estimated at 15,000,000 inhabitants with fifty two per cent women and forty eight per cent men, of whom 48.2 per cent live in urban areas and 51.8 per cent in rural zones (DSCN, 1998). Women in the reproductive age constitute twenty three per cent of the population, while the children from zero to five years old constitute eighteen per cent. The total fertility rate is estimated at 5.2 children per woman of fifteen to forty nine years old and corresponds to a crude birthrate of about 3.7 per cent. The illiteracy rate is twenty four for the adult population, twenty eight per cent for women and fifteen per cent for men (EDSC-II, 1998).

Since the end of the eighties, the country has experienced an economic crisis characterized by a decreasing economic growth. This has been coupled with budget cuts and reduced public investments in the social sector, which has led to an increased level of poverty. Indeed, between 1986 and 1988 real GDP decreased by eleven per cent, while gross domestic investment and consumption went down by thirty-eight per cent and nine per cent, respectively. The unemployment rate was estimated at seventeen per cent (DSCN, 1998). As regards well-being, the DSCN estimated the incidence of poverty at 50.52 per cent using the Cameroonian 1996 household budget survey (ECAM). Kamgnia and Timnou (2000) determined a poverty incidence rate of 52.8 per cent using the food energy intake approach, while Fambon *et al.*, (2000) obtained a rate of sixty five per cent, using the cost of basic needs approach. With a per capita GNP that decreased from US $1010 in 1988 to $680 in 1994, the country now belongs to the group of low-income countries (MSP, 1999).

The bulk of the sanitary directorate comprises 1491 healthcare units, of which 392 are privately owned. According to UNICEF (1998), the medical coverage of the country by the public sector is thirty six per cent, private formal health centers coverage is seventeen per cent while that for private informal centers is fourteen per cent. Since the WHO recommends allocation of about ten per cent of the annual budget towards the health sector, one would say that the financing of the health sector in Cameroon is still too low. Indeed, out of the 173 billion spent on healthcare in Cameroon in 1996, seventy three per cent were incurred by the households themselves (DSCN; 1996). In fact, the households participate in the financing of healthcare in the form of fees and other consultation related costs, which contradicts the nationwide efforts at alleviating poverty. The reduced level of investment in the public health sector tends to hamper the performance of the various programs for the control of endemic diseases that require large scale distribution of pharmaceutical products in the community.

The supply and distribution of drugs and of other pharmaceutical products undertaken by the National Center for Essential Drugs Supply (NCEDS)[1], and the wholesale-distributors. The drugs and pharmaceutical products

[1] Stands for the acronym CENAME, that is, « Centrale Nationale d'Approvisionnement en Médicaments Essentiels ».

are sourced from the pharmaceutical industries, both locally based (10%) and foreign ones (90%) (MSP, 2000). The NCEDS ensures the availability of generic drugs to its principal customers who are: Provincial Pharmaceutical Centers, General Hospitals and Purchasing Centers that are the main suppliers of denominational medical centers as well as the non-lucrative undenominational ones. The wholesale-distributors supply private pharmacies, and also on a non-conventional basis, the private health centers, the general and central hospitals. However, the tendency is towards the development of some parallel, illicit and informal sale networks of drugs and pharmaceutical products, along with self-medication and the resort to traditional medicine.

5.1.2 The burden of malaria

Despite the partial success of the eradication efforts over the sixties and the malaria control strategies of the eighties, this endemic disease still remains a social and economic burden and a serious public health problem in Africa in the 21st century.

5.1.3 The effects of malaria in the world

Malaria is one of the most ravaging vectorial diseases in the world. Each year, some forty one per cent (2.3 billion) of the world population is at the risk of infection by plasmodium. There are between 300 and 500 million of malaria cases and 1.5 to 2.7 millions of malaria related deaths per year (Kassankogno, 1999a)[2]. Malaria is particularly prevalent among the poor (Gbary, 1999). However, more than eighty per cent of the clinical cases and approximately ninety-five per cent of malaria related deaths in the world are specific to Africa. Indeed, approximately ninety per cent of the African population lives in zones of high endemicity or those at the risk of epidemic malaria, i.e are characterized by a malaria incidence of about 700 cases in 1000 inhabitants (Magda, 1999)[3].

It is estimated that forty per cent to fifty per cent of internal admissions in healthcare centers in Africa are malaria related, which adds up to forty per

---

2. As stated by Maurice (1992), with 270 million of infected individuals, 110 million of new cases recorded each year, 1 to 2 million of annual deaths (notably among children) and about 3 billion individuals (more than 40% of the world population) at a risk of malaria infection in more than 100 countries, malaria stands out as the most devastating tropical disease.

3. The striking fact is that African countries make the bulk of countries that are not included in the WHO's global strategy for malaria control (WHO; 1993).

cent of the expenditures on public health and constitutes up to fifty per cent of the external consultations in the infected zones. Overall, one could consider malaria as one of the major causes of misery, poverty and inequality in Africa. Indeed, each episode of malaria corresponds to one to three days lost from work for an adult in Nigeria, two to four days lost from work in Kenya and nineteen days lost from work in Burkina Faso, accounting for eight per cent of decreases in the labor force in Nigeria and two per cent to six per cent in Kenya.

The economic costs (direct and indirect) associated with malaria worldwide were estimated at 2 billion US dollars in 1997 and at US3.6 billion dollars in year 2000 (Kassankogno, 1999a, 1999b). As far as Africa is concerned, Gallup and Sachs (2000) point out that its GDP would have been higher by thirty two per cent, say by US 100 billion dollars, over its current level, if malaria had been eradicated thirty five years ago. Accordingly, malaria systematically slows down the annual growth of the GNP by 1.3 per cent in countries of endemic malaria, which are among the poorest in the world. Moreover, an infected household on average devotes more than one quarter of its income to malaria treatment, while also having to face prevention expenses as well as opportunity costs of seeking care. Malaria compromises the education of youngsters in areas of high malaria endemicity and constitutes one of the primary causes of school absenteeism.

5.1.4 The effects of malaria in Cameroon

Malaria is a major public health problem both in terms of morbidity and mortality in Cameroon. As regards morbidity, two million[4] cases of malaria are reported each year by medical centers. According to Soula *et al.*, (2001), although statistics are difficult to establish for such a complex pathology, one could say that it is responsible for thirty to fifty per cent of reported medical consultations; twenty per cent of the total hospital admissions; and twenty five to forty-five per cent of the cases of deaths among children of zero to five years old.

4. Such a figure could be considered as an underestimation of the true rate. Indeed, even if all the cases are not treated in healthcare centers, each one of the 15 million Cameroonians faces at least one malaria episode each year.

Malaria remains a real concern at all community levels, especially due to the resistance of its principal vector Plasmodium falciparum to some of the drugs, notably chloroquine,[5] which is the most commonly used drug in the treatment of malaria in Cameroon. In effect, although malaria is attributed to 4 species of plasmodium, namely P. falciparum, P. vivax, P. ovale and P. malariae, Plasmodium falciparum stands out as the most death related[6] vector, since it is responsible for the most pernicious form of malaria. More specifically, malaria cases due to plasmodium in Cameroon are distributed in terms of P. falciparum (96%), P. malariae (3%), and P. ovale (1%). While the coastal zone[7] stands out as the high resistance zone of P. falciparum to chloroquine (18 to 30%), the savannah zone is a low resistance zone (6 to 15%). Moreover, malaria is an economic burden in Cameroon. According to Soula *et al.,* (2000), it is responsible for seventy-five per cent of days lost from work (days off due to illness), accounting for forty per cent of the yearly expenditures of households on health care.

As far as malaria control is concerned, the national program conforms to the principles of the global initiative of "Roll Back Malaria" in terms of the following control strategies:

- Provision of treatment for complaints of malaria, in terms of an early diagnosis followed by a rapid and appropriate treatment of benign cases of malaria either at home or at healthcare centers, and the treatment of most serious cases exclusively in the medical centers;
- Prevention of the disease; what is done in terms of the fight against mosquitoes responsible for the transmission of the disease, through: (i) hygiene and the cleanliness of the immediate surroundings of the houses, and (ii) household-based protection measures (fences at the windows, bed nets and insecticide-treated curtains, etc.); and
- Information, education and communication on malaria, its causes, consequences, treatment and prevention.

---

5. Following the historical analysis done on the drug-resistance by Hengy (1988), although the first signs of the resistance were determined in 1960, resistance in Cameroon was detected in 1985, and that of Yaoundé in 1986.
6. P. vivax is the most popular form, while P. ovale and P. malariae are rather rare (Maurice; 1992).
7. The first cases of resistance in Central Africa were identified in the coastal zone (Hengy, (1988).

The implementation of strategies for malaria control rests on the solution to the following three challenges. First, malaria, considered for a long time as a consequence of poverty, is also a major cause of poverty and its prevention remains a significant component of the fight against poverty. From this point of view, reducing import taxes and custom duties on bed nets and other products such as insecticides and anti-malarial drugs would render the strategies of the fight against malaria more accessible to all households in the communities. Second, the cheapest anti-malarial drug, chloroquine, quickly loses its effectiveness in most of the health districts or in the communities with high malaria endemicity. In Cameroon, malaria is resistant to the four most widespread drugs for its treatment in a number of health districts. Thirdly, deficiencies in the healthcare systems, coupled with malaria resistance to treatment drugs, along with the migration of the populations, the climatic change and the uncontrolled development activities, contribute to the rise in malaria incidence.

5.1.5 The control of malaria

Hamadicko (1990) conceives the fight against malaria as having two components: the fight against the parasite hosted by a sick person and the vectorial fight. However, according to Chinmoun (1997), the anti-malarial fight is based on an interdisciplinary strategy comprising a curative treatment, the control of the anopheles mosquitoes, and prevention. Whatever the strategy, the fight against the parasite calls for the use of anti-malarial drugs, either for a curative treatment or for a radical treatment[8]. The principal curative drugs are either of the schizontocides group (drugs acting on the asexual erythrocyte form of plasmodium) such as quinine and amino-4-quinolines, or of the group of the gametocytocides group. However, the most commonly used drugs are those of the first group which happen to be less toxic. As far as the anti-vectorial fight is concerned, its aim is to eradicate the vectorial mosquitoes and their larval lodgings in order to reduce, and prevent the transmission of the disease, using either collective means or household specific means. Unfortunately, the effectiveness of the anti-vectorial control is strongly compromised by an insufficient knowledge of the ecology of the vectors, which limits the choice of the methods to be used (Chinmoun, 1997), while the fight against the parasite is constrained by the problem of drug-resistance.

8. Here, Hamadicko refers to André *et al.*, (1980).

Considering the challenges thus highlighted and the need to improve the strategies for malaria control, it becomes necessary to assess the patterns of the demand for malaria control products and services in Cameroon. This is an analysis of a particular case of an urban community of Yaoundé that is considered as a zone of hypo-endemicity (Hamadicko, 1990).

5.2 Objectives and Hypotheses of the Study

5.2.1 Objectives of the study

The general objective of this study was to provide some relevant statistics on the characteristics of the demand for malaria control products (drugs, insecticides and bed nets) in four health districts in the urban community of Yaoundé, Cameroon. The specific objectives were to:

(i) Determine the degree of awareness about malaria and the use of anti-malarial drugs, insecticides and bed nets in the control and/or prevention of malaria;
(ii) Identify the socioeconomic factors that determine the choice of malaria service providers, and sources of drugs;
and
(ii) Make policy recommendations on actions or strategies necessary to enhance the accessibility of malaria control products in the study area.

5.2.2 Research hypotheses

The Main Hypothesis: Malaria control products have substitutes or complements whose prices are major determinants of demand for pharmaceutical products.

The Secondary Hypothesis 1: Consumers of healthcare services have limited information about malaria, and this situation favors supplier inducement of the demand for malaria control products and services.

The Secondary Hypothesis 2: Low-income malaria patients frequently resort to self-medication. Malaria control products are mainly reputation goods whose demand is a function of the information given by family members, friends and neighbors. This information helps consumers to select among the various types of products available in pharmaceutical markets.

5.3 Methodology of the Study

Three significant elements of the methodological aspect of the study are: the survey, the analysis of the collected data and the modelling and estimation of demand for pharmaceuticals. The design of a new survey proved to be necessary because the existing data bases, ECAM-96, and EDS-98, were carried out to satisfy objectives that are very different from those of the current study. Indeed, the relevant variables for evaluation of the state of awareness about malaria and the use of anti-malarial drugs were not included in those databases. In this study, contrary to the logic that suggests that data should be collected in order to validate a given model, we started instead with data concerns, followed by analytical techniques and finally, considered the demand models that needed estimation.

5.3.1 Target populations, areas of the study and survey methods

The target population of the study involved households in four health districts (Biyem-Assi, Cite Verte, Djoungolo and Nkoldongo) in the urban community of Yaoundé in Cameroon. The observation units were the household heads or their spouses present in the community on the day of the investigation.

To ensure representativeness of the sample, a random sampling technique was used. More specifically, a three-stage sampling exercise was undertaken. Each health district was divided into clusters according to its demographic importance. In the first stage, a random sample of clusters was selected. In the second stage, households were selected from each one of the selected clusters. In the third stage, the household heads or their spouses were randomly selected from the selected households. The selection of the first household in the sample was randomly done. The selection procedure was as follows: the center of each cluster was identified and the nearest intersection to that center was taken as the starting point for the investigator. Moving from that center, the investigator randomly determined the path to follow and proceeded in the same way to determine the first household to sample. Then he moved gradually until he obtained the required number of respondents for the considered cluster.

5.3.2 The sample size

The plan of action for malaria control in Cameroon for 2000–2001 indicates that malaria accounts for fifty per cent of the medical consultations in

Cameroon. Based on that information and on the significant proportion of malaria infected households, it appeared necessary to define a large sample in order to secure a high proportion of households having had at least a malaria episode during the twelve months prior to the survey. The number of such individuals should be large enough to guarantee the reliability of the statistical analysis to be made. Hence, the size of the sample of households was calculated using the following formula[9]:

$$n = \frac{Z^2 \pi (1 - \pi)}{d^2}$$

where,

n = size of the sample of households in the urban community of Yaoundé;

Z = value of the standard normal deviate, determined as 1.96 for a ninety-five per cent degree of confidence, a value that we rounded to two in the present study;

π = indicator of prevalence of malaria in the medical consultations in Cameroon. This proportion is estimated at fifty per cent, say 0.50;

d = allowed margin of error for a degree of accuracy or confidence interval estimated at ninety-five per cent; defined at five per cent, that is, 0.05.

Hence given a value of the indicator of prevalence estimated at 0.50, a Z value set equal to two, and a degree of accuracy of 0.95; the sample size was determined as:

$$n = \frac{(2^2)(0.50)(0.50)}{(0.50)^2}$$

which gives, n = 400 households.

---

9. This is derived from Miller and Freund (1985), *Probability and Statistics for Engineers,* third edition, Prentice-Hall.

5.3.3 Data collection

Materials and methods

The data was collected based on a pre-coded and structured[10] questionnaire. In order to guarantee the confidentiality of the revealed information, the questionnaire was made anonymous. The final version of the questionnaire was drawn after its pre-testing on some households selected from a sample neighborhoods. In each area, the data were collected using individual interviews. The mode of administration of the questionnaires was direct. Answers provided by a respondent were collected by an enumerator and registered on an individual questionnaire for each selected household. The language used for the interview was French.

Survey agents

Two categories of personnel were involved in the survey: enumerators and supervisors. The enumerators were in charge of the direct collection of the data in the field while the supervisors were in charge of the allocation of the functions between the various enumerators, the supervision, and the daily checking of their work.

Two teams of twelve investigators (both males and females) and two supervisors undertook the fieldwork. The investigators and interviewers were recruited from among the doctorate students majoring in public health and some students in social sciences based on their experience in data collection, investigation and their ability to express themselves in French. They were given an additional training centered on the techniques of data gathering and the filling of questionnaires. The training was structured around the following points: (i) the context of the study and presentation of the project; (ii) malaria and its socio-economic burden in Africa and in Cameroon; (iii) scientific objectives of the investigation and its usefulness for public health; (iv) methodology of the investigation; (v) techniques of filling the questionnaires; and (vi) simulation of interviews.

---

[10]. Overall, the questionnaire was structured to comprise: i) a front page; ii) a section on the identification of the area of the survey; iii) a section on the awareness about malaria and patients' therapeutic behavior, and iv) a section on the prevention of malaria and awareness about insecticide-treated bed nets.

Each enumerator and supervisor was given a card entitled "guide to the enumerator and supervisor", which displayed the instructions to be used in field research.

The analysis of data

After editing the data using Epi Info version 6.04, the descriptive analysis of the data was done on SPSS, while estimations of the specified models were performed using STATA.

5.3.4 The determinants of demand for malaria control products and services

The design of malaria control policies requires, among others, the knowledge of the determinants of the demand for malaria control products and services. These can be identified as factors influencing, either the quantities demanded, or the probability that the household demands a given malaria control product or service. We chose to analyze the factors that determine (i) the probability that an individual demands malaria drugs irrespective of source (ii) the probability that the individual resorts to a particular drug source, and (iii) the probability that an individual visits a service provider.

Although a number of anti-malaria drugs are being used in the urban community of Yaoundé, the most commonly used ones are quinine, chloroquine and amodiaquine. In collecting the necessary data for the analysis, individuals were asked if they took a specific drug or not, rather than if they chose to take it over the other drugs. As far as the sources of drugs are concerned, the survey specified four categories: (i) pharmacies, (ii) street vendors, (iii) public hospitals, and (iv) private hospitals. However, in analyzing the individuals' choice of the facility they acquired the drugs from, we grouped facilities into two categories: the informal facilities, consisting of street vendors and the formal drug facilities consisting of pharmacies and hospitals, either public or private. As regards service types, these comprised self-medication, modern medicine and traditional medicine, which we grouped into self-medication (including traditional medicine) and modern services.

An individual resorting to self-medication can walk into a pharmacy and obtain the product that he wishes to take. However, it is likely that the acquisition of the products from the pharmacy or from the public or private hospital, is mainly done by those individuals who resort to the formal healthcare system; those resorting to self-medication tend to acquire drugs from street vendors.

On the modeling side, a qualitative binary dependent variable was defined in each one of the three decisions being analyzed: for drug use (equals 1 if the considered drug was being used and 0 for other types of drugs[11]), a drug source (equals 1 if modern facility and 0 for street vendors), and the provision of malaria services (equals 1 if hospital service was used and 0 for self-medication). Appropriate models in these situations are the Probits and Logits[12]. Based on the fact that the three decisions were independently taken, three separate Probit models were analyzed, based on the following general considerations.

All consumers were assumed to possess utility functions $U = U(x_1, x_2, \ldots, x_k)$ which are differentiable everywhere, and which are strictly increasing $(U'_j > 0, I = 1, 2, \ldots, k)$ and strictly quasi-concave. The standard microeconomic model defines the X_js as goods and services, while Lancaster (1966) presents them as satisfactions produced by the individuals from the combination of the specified goods and services. The utilities underlying Lancaster's analysis could be considered when modeling the demand for health services for which degrees of satisfaction rather than quantity consumed are relevant.

In each one of the above three decisions (choice of malaria treatment, service provider on the one part, and malaria drug source on the other part), one could postulate the existence of a random utility U_j, (j = 0, 1) such that

$$U_1 = Z_1\beta + \varepsilon_1$$

and $$U_0 = Z_0\beta + \varepsilon_0,$$

---

11. Such a specification required an additional coding of the data to allow a given drug to be evaluated against the other ones.

12. While the Probit model is based on the hypothesis of a normal distribution, the Logit model assumes a logistic distribution. The two distributions differ only at their tails, and because the logistic distribution has a variance of $\pi^2/3$, the estimates of the coefficients from the Logit model are roughly a factor $\pi/\sqrt{3}$ larger than those obtained from the Probit model (Verbeek, 2000).

where, U_1 and U_0 are the utilities derived from using the chosen alternative, and that derived from the alternative mode, respectively. Z_1 and Z_0 are matrices of characteristics specific to the respective alternatives. The observed choice between the two alternatives depends on whichever of the alternatives provides the greater utility. In other words, the claim is as follows;

$$Y = 1 \text{ if } U_1 > U_0$$
and
$$Y = 0 \text{ if } U_1 < U_0$$

Thus, *the probability that* $Y = 1$ could be expressed as:

$$\begin{aligned} Prob\ (U_1 > U_0) &= Prob\ (Z_1\beta + \varepsilon_1 > Z_0\beta + \varepsilon_0) \\ &= Prob\ (\varepsilon_1 - \varepsilon_0 > Z_0\beta - Z_1\beta) \\ &= Prob\ (\varepsilon > -X\beta) \end{aligned}$$

Under a hypothesis of a normal distribution, the symmetry of the distribution allows us to verify that

$$Prob\ (U_1 > U_0) = Prob\ (\varepsilon < X\beta) = F(X\beta).$$

Finally, we may state that

$$Prob(y_i = 1) = \int_{-\infty}^{X\beta} \phi(t)dt = \Phi(X\beta).$$

In such a specification, ε is a vector of components unobserved by the researcher, although those might be known to the individual in question. From a statistical point of view, ε would be considered as a random "noise", which is normally distributed. *X* defines a matrix of explanatory variables (relative to either one of the two alternatives, that is, a pool of elements of Z_1 and Z_0).

5.3.5 Economic variables

The "economic variables" that were analyzed comprised mainly the prices of drugs, and the cost of healthcare. The effect of individuals' income could have been investigated, but few respondents revealed their income during the survey.

"Individual level variables", included variables such as a dummy for the sex of the household head, four dummies for the level of education (primary, secondary O-Level, secondary A-level, university), two dummies for the religion of the household head (Christian and Muslim), age groups of the household head, four dummies for the socio-professional category of the household head (administrative, agriculture, laborer, and tradesman), and the average number of malaria episodes incurred by the household head, that is, the number of malaria attacks.

"Mode of treatment" was defined as a dummy specific to hospital, against a self-medication alternative, which included traditional practitioner).

"Types of drugs" involved two dummies for chloroquine against the other medicines, and for quinine against the other drugs.

Household level determinants, were the number of young children (0 to 5 years old), number of older children and number of malaria cases.

An individual must first decide to seek treatment before choosing the service and/or the pharmaceutical product to use. Thus, a conditional logit model would have been appropriate in each one of the three cases of decisions analyzed. However, we decided to consider only the persons who treated themselves for malaria attacks. Considering only those persons who treated themselves might give rise to a problem of sample selection bias and therefore require use of the Heckman correction method. Nevertheless, we think that consistent estimates can be obtained without going through the Heckman (1979) correction[13] method given that only a few respondents (2%) did not treat themselves.

Another problem that could have affected the quality of the estimation is the possible interrelation among the three decisions, especially between the choice of service provider and that of drug use. However, the questionnaire was constructed such that the decisions were taken independently, and thus can be analyzed using independent Probit models.

---

[13]. The Heckman correction method or Heckit method or Heckman's lambda is a two stage estimation procedure. In the current case, in the first stage, a model of the decision to self-treat would have been estimated in order to obtain the estimated odds. In the second stage, specifying the estimated odds as an additional explanatory variable in either of the analyzed models would have resulted in consistent estimates of the coefficients of those models.

5.4 Findings

This sub-section presents sample statistics and estimation results from various models of demand for malaria treatments and prevention. Table 5.1 shows main socio-economic characteristics of the sample households.

5.4.1 The socio-demographic characteristics of the households

The aim at this point is to present the major socio-demographic characteristics of the individuals that have been successfully surveyed during the current study. The various characteristics are presented in table 5.1.

As shown in table 5.1, 400 households (of which 111 from Cite Verte, 126 from Djoungolo, sixty three from Nkol Ndongo and 100 from Biyem-Assi) were successfully surveyed. Overall, the households are proportionally distributed over the four health districts considered in the study. However, the distribution of the respondents by zone of residence, irrespective of the areas of study, is rather unequal as more than three quarters (75%) of the households live in the popular urban zones.

Concerning the age structure of the respondents, no significant difference is observed over the health districts. The age distribution indicates a mean age of thirty five years among the respondents. The median age is thirty three years for all the areas. According to the status of a individual in the household, it appears that the household heads (62%) are more represented than their spouses (38%). The analysis by sex shows that there are more males (59%) than females (41%), which is primarily due to the fact that the survey was conducted in an urban area where the tendencies are such that the proportion of males outweighs that of females. Overall, the average size of the households is 6.44, compared with a median of six individuals across the four districts.

As regards the occupation of the respondents, the most common categories are: tradesmen (26%), unemployed (23%), civil servants and workers of the private sector (17% and 13%) respectively; while farmers (3%) are under-represented. Such a tendency remains the same when the distribution is defined according to areas of residence.

Concerning the number of children (0–5 years) in the household, it appears that the majority (53%) of the respondents do not have children of this age interval in their households; a little more than one individual out of five (26%) have a child, and one out of four (22%) has two children and more. As regards the number of pregnant women in the household, the great majority of the respondents (89%) declared that there was no pregnant woman in their households. Those that declared having at least one pregnant woman in their households account for nine per cent of the respondents.

With respect to the level of education, the majority (97%) of the respondents can read and write, being almost equally distributed over the four educational categories: primary school (21%), secondary school O-level (27%), secondary school A-level (27%), and university (21%). As regards religion, Christians make up the greatest percentage (73%), followed by Muslims (23%), and others (5%).

5.4.2 Awareness of malaria

The objective of this subsection is to describe the extent of awareness about the symptoms and modes of transmission of malaria (Table 5.2). The degree of awareness about malaria depends on exposure to information on malaria.

5.4.3 Knowledge about the symptoms of malaria

The data relating to the knowledge about the symptoms of malaria are presented in table 5.2. Overall, only a small proportion (< 1%) of the respondents did not indicate a symptom of malaria. Nearly all the respondents (99.8%) had already heard about malaria. Prior to this survey. Moreover, forty three per cent said there is a local name to describe this disease. The most commonly known symptoms among the respondents, either male or female were: fever (61.67%), headaches (57.78%), feeling cold (43.11%), and to a lesser extent, tiredness (37.42%).

Thus, more than six respondents out of ten (61.67%) knew that fever is the major symptom of malaria. Nevertheless, other symptoms were referred to by the respondents: headaches (57.78%), feeling cold (43.11%), tiredness (37.42%), aches (29.34%), lack of appetite (20.66%), and vomiting (23.05%). This reveals that the signs of severe malaria were not well known by the sample population. However, the average individual was

Table 5.1 Socio-demographic characteristics of the households

Area of the Study and Characteristics of the Households	Cite-Verte	Djoun-golo	Nkol-Ndongo	Biyem-Assi	Total
Size of the Household					
Mean	5.48	6.57	6.79	7.42	6.44
Median	5	6	6	6	6
Age of the Respondent (years)					
Mean	31.87	36.91	33.51	38.95	34.88
Median	30.50	36	32	37	33
Type of Residential area (%)					
Urban	22	12.6	6.3	4	12
Urban Commercial	10.8	16.67	9.5	7	11.5
Urban Popular	64.86	70.63	79.36	88	74.75
Rural	2.70	0	4.76	1	1.75
Sex of respondent (%)					
Male	60.36	57.14	73	51	59
Female	39.64	42.85	27	49	41
Status in the Household (%)					
Household Head	67.56	61.11	82.54	45	62.25
Spouse	32.43	38.89	17.46	55	37.75
Occupation of the Respondent (%)					
Unemployed	17.39	25.24	18.52	28.98	22.64
Laborer of the Private Sector	11.95	14.56	14.81	8.69	12.57
Civil Servant	18.47	11.65	16.66	23.18	16.98
Administrative of the Private Sector	4.34	2.91	5.55	5.79	4.40
Administrative of the Public Sector	5.34	5.82	5.55	5.79	4.40

Continued

Table 5.1 *(continued)*

Area of the Study and Characteristics of the Households	Cite-Verte	Djoun-golo	Nkol-Ndongo	Biyem-Assi	Total
Tradesmen of the Informal Sector	5.43	11.65	11.11	4.35	8.17
Tradesmen of the Formal Sector	33.69	26.21	22.22	20.29	26.41
Farmer	3.26	1.94	5.55	2.89	3.14
Education of the respondent (%)					
Illiterate	5.45	4	1.58	1	3.26
Primary	22.72	28	15.87	14	21.10
Secondary O-level	24.54	29.6	30.16	26	27.39
Secondary A-level	28.18	22.4	33.33	27	26.88
University	19.09	16	19.05	32	21.36
Religion of the respondent (%)					
Christian	66.05	74.60	81.96	71.43	72.59
Muslem	32.11	20.69	8.19	23.47	22.59
Traditional Religion	1.83	4.76	9.84	5.10	4.82
Total	**111**	**126**	**63**	**100**	**400**

Source: Constructed by the author based on the survey data.

aware of the most commonly known symptom of malaria, namely, fever. Indeed, following the description of Nájera *et al.,* (1992), the principal symptom of malaria is fever; the other signs, such as weakness, convulsion, jaundice, giddiness, hypoglycemia, spontaneous bleeding, and pulmonary edema are signs of severity. Such signs are detected clinically and thus cannot be easily known by the individuals.

Knowledge about the modes of transmission of malaria

One of the objectives of this study was to determine the proportion of respondents who had correct knowledge about modes of transmission of malaria. Hence, the study was interested in those who indicated mosquito bites as the major mode of transmission of the disease. As to the question

Table 5.2 Distribution (%) of the households according to the symptoms of malaria that they knew

Area of the Study and Knowledge about the Symptoms	Cité-Verte	Djoun-golo	Nkol-Ndongo	Biyem-Assi	Total
Has Heard About Malaria	99	100	100	100	99.7
Does not Know					
Fever	59.57	59.81	63.79	65.33	61.67
Feeling Cold	43.62	38.32	51.72	42.67	43.11
Headache	62.76	47.66	68.96	57.33	57.78
Coca Cola Colored Urine	1.06	1.86	3.45	5.33	2.69
Vomiting	19.14	20.56	24.14	30.67	23.05
Diarrhoea	4.25	7.47	3.44	6.67	5.69
Tiredness	45.74	26.17	34.48	45.33	37.42
Lack of Appetite	13.82	19.62	25.86	26.67	20.66
Aches	25.53	33.64	36.21	22.67	29.34
Jaundice	7.44	6.54	3.45	4.00	5.69
Giddiness	6.38	3.74	5.17	9.33	5.99
Abdominal Pains	5.32	3.74	6.89	1.33	4.19
Nausea	5.32	5.61	3.45	1.33	4.19
Discomfort	9.57	3.74	6.89	5.33	6.29
Mouth Herpesus	1.06	1.87	1.72	1.33	1.49
Convulsions	4.25	1.87	8.62	4.00	4.19
Anemia	9.57	3.74	3.45	4.00	5.38
Coma	2.13	1.86	3.45	2.67	2.29
Obnubilation/Confusion	1.06	0.00	0.00	0.00	0.29
Prostration	1.06	0.00	0.00	0.00	0.29
Kidney Failure	2.13	0.00	01.72	0.00	0.59
Hypoglycemia	1.06	0.93	–	0.00	0.89
Total	**94**	**107**	**58**	**75**	**334**

Source: Compiled by the author based on the survey data.

of knowledge about the modes of transmission of malaria, about one respondent in twelve (8%) did not indicate any mode of transmission. However, twenty five per cent of the females indicated that they did not know any mode of transmission, while the percentage was twenty one per cent among the males. Nonetheless, one should note that the majority (79%) of the respondents, mostly males (68%), compared to females (62%) indicated mosquito bites as the main mode of transmission of malaria. This category of respondents corresponds to about one respondent in five, as shown in table 5.3.

Table 5.3 Distribution of the households according to the mode of transmission of malaria

Mode of Transmission	Percentages of Respondents
Does not Know	8.8
Working under the Sun	3.3
Staying Under the Rain	10.8
Catching Cold	15.8
Drinking Salty water	9.0
Contact with Malarious Persons	1.8
Mosquito Bites	79.0
Other	12.5

Source: Compiled by the author based on the survey data.

5.4.4 Perception about the risk of malaria

Perception about the risk of contracting malaria: The objective here was to assess the respondents' perception about the risk of catching malaria, as well as their perception about the risk that the most vulnerable groups, in particular children (0–5 years), would catch the disease. Indeed, the perception of the respondents about the risk of children (0–5 years) contracting malaria would help to correctly assess their knowledge about the disease.

Table 5.4 presents the distribution of the respondents according to their opinion about the risk that children of their household would catch malaria.

It appears from the table that the proportion of the respondents is negatively correlated with their perception about the risk that children (0–5 years) would catch malaria. The table shows that children of less than five years are more at risk of malaria. More specifically, the data indicates that children of less than five years old (33.6%), pregnant women (24.73%) and everyone (20.92%) are at greater risk of catching malaria. Thus, in each household, eight-two per cent of the identified cases of malaria concerned the children of less than five years old (Table 5.5).

Table 5.4 Distribution (%) of respondents according to their perception of the group most vulnerable to malaria

Area of the Study and Group at Risk of Malaria	Cité-Verte	Djoun-golo	Nkol-Ndongo	Biyem-Assi	Total
Children < 5 Years	10.05	8.54	4.52	10.05	33.16
Pregnant Women	6.12	7.71	3.72	7.18	24.73
Everyone	6.52	6.25	3.53	4.62	20.92

Note: The question was asked to determine if the group in question could catch malaria (very easily, easily, rarely, not at all).

Source: Compiled by the author based on the survey data.

In general, ninety-seven per cent of the respondents think that people can die of malaria. Concerning their backgrounds with respect to malaria, the great majority of the respondents (90.7%) stated that they had at least one episode of malaria during the last twelve months preceding the survey. The results also show that children at zero to five years old are among the

Table 5.5 Cases of malaria that involved children of less than 5 years old

Area of the Study Cases of Malaria	Cité-Verte	Djoun-golo	Nkol-Ndongo	Biyem-Assi	Total
Children < 5 Years	82.10	80.73	79.31	85.89	82.05
Total	**95**	**109**	**58**	**78**	**340**

Source: Compiled by the author based on the survey data.

people in their households who suffered most from malaria during the twelve months preceding the investigation. In fact, the majority of the respondents indicated that it is easy to catch malaria. As regards the group that is at risk of malaria "everyone" (54.89%) comes first, followed by "pregnant women" (52.92%), and finally "children of less than five years" (47.49%).

Exposure of the households to malaria risks during the twelve months preceeding the survey: The exposure of the respondents to malaria is measured here by the individual having ever had malaria during the entire life and by the number of episodes of malaria that the respondent had during the twelve months before the survey.

It emerges from the analysis that nearly all the respondents (94%) stated that they had had malaria before the survey. The groups at the greatest risk are: people above age of forty years, and persons living in the popular zones. Concerning the other social groups, it appears that in the popular urban areas, females (96%) and unemployed (95%), constituted the majority of those who declared as having had malaria. The group of those who did not have malaria during the past twelve months (33%) was made up of young people, people living in residential areas (39%), males (38%), household heads (35%), and the unemployed (40%).

Figure 5.1 Distribution of households according to modes of treatment

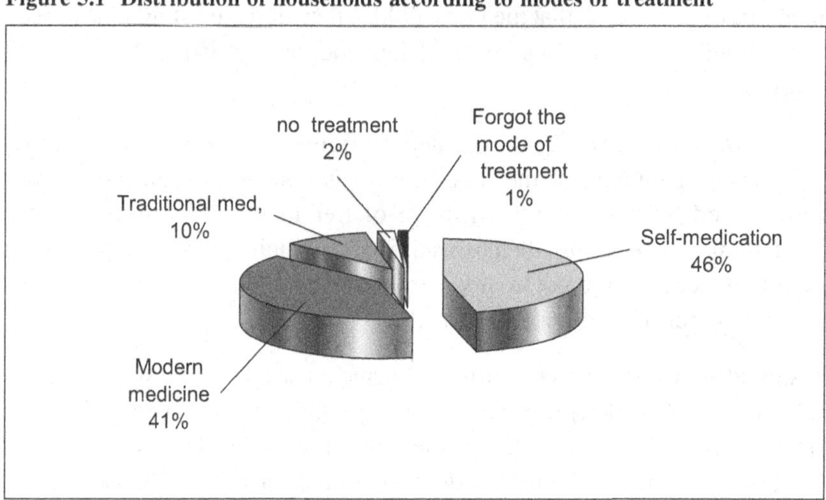

Source: Constructed by the author based on the survey data.

Figure 5.2 Distribution of households according to the type of anti-malarial drugs used

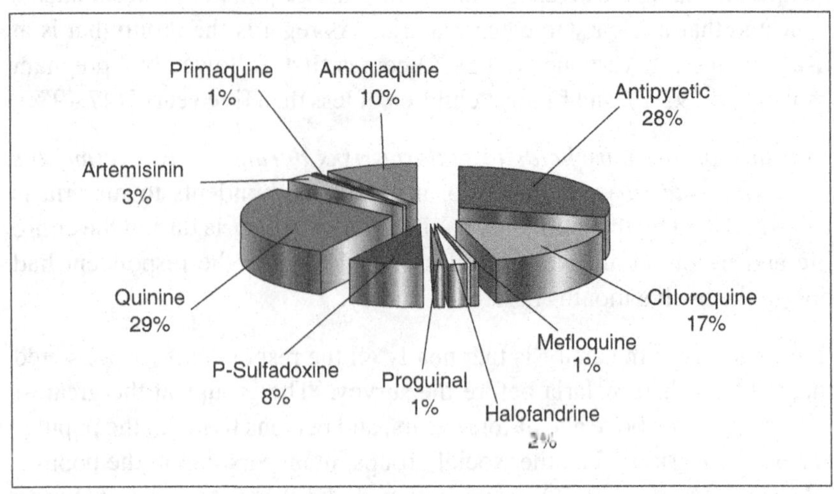

Source: Constructed by the author based on the survey data.

5.4.5 Therapeutic behavior and use of malaria control products

The aim here is to assess the behavior of the households with respect to the fight against the vector that is hosted by the human being and the methods of prevention that the households knew or were using. The modes of treatment, types of drugs used and their sources are also analyzed in this section.

The modes of treatment: As revealed by figure 5.1, as far as the care of the various members of the household was concerned, self-medication represented the most common mode of treatment (46%), followed by modern medicine (41%), then by traditional medicine (10%); only two per cent of the cases were not treated, and only one per cent of patients could not remember the mode of treatment.

It should be noted that the results of the current study are in line with those of Soula *et al.*, (2000) as regards the importance of self-medication and modern medicine. However, Soula *et al,* found that modern medicine ranked first as the preferred mode of treatment in 1997. The two years, 1997 and 2001, coincide with the period of economic recovery in Cameroon.

Yet, given that the effects of the economic crisis became less severe during the second half of the nineties, one would have expected that in 2001 more households would have resorted to modern medicine. That, however was not the case. In fact, Soula *et al.,* (2000) attributed the importance of self-medication to the negative effects of high costs of consultation, the over-prescriptions, and the practices of parallel sales in the medical centers. Those practices became the rule rather than the exception in 2001 as efforts made by the Government to increase the wages in the public sector in 2000 led to the increase in prices in many sectors, of which the modern healthcare sector was one. The issue here was to investigate the types of drugs used by the households during this period.

Drugs use: In terms of drugs used, quinine ranked first, along with the antipyretic drugs[14] (figure 5.2). Chloroquine occupies the second position among the anti-malarial drugs, which is in conformity with findings of Hengy *et al.,* (1988). Chloroquine keeps its position of a drug of first choice, particularly in the presumptive treatment of malaria attacks. Moreover, the classification of the products used by the respondents generally follows that of modes of treatment identified by Hengy *et al.* Indeed, whereas those two products (quinine and chloroquine) are financially more accessible than products like halofandrine, there was a tendency to discourage amodiaquine, because of its being associated with cases of agranulocytose and of hepatitis which, in the majority of the cases leads to death (Chinmoun, 1997).

As for proguanil, Chinmoun (1997) indicates that its use in a strategy of mass treatment quickly leads to the appearance of drug-resistance of P. falciparum and P. vivax, yet it does not prevent malaria attacks. Rather, proguanil appears essential in preventive treatment of feverish attacks[15]. Following Basco (2001), mefloquine, artemisinin and their various derivatives are being introduced in Cameroon and thus might not be well known by the sample population. This explains the low proportions of respondents who used those drugs.

---

[14] The association of quinine with the antipyretics (non-anti-malarial drugs) is necessary in cases of malaria coupled with fever and headaches.

[15] That does not mean that quinine is harmless. Indeed, Chinmoun (1997) indicates, among other cardio-vascular effects, side effects such as hemoglobin, uric fever and some heartburns.

However, in the face of risk of resistance to chloroquine drug-resistance, new tendency in Central Africa is towards drug combination therapies against malaria instead of monotherapies, especially those based on chloroquine[16]. One such combination includes artemether-lumefantrine, artesunate and amodiaquine[17]. The various anti-malarial drugs are shown in appendix tables 5.AI–5.A13.

Sources of drugs: The distribution of the households according to sources of pharmaceutical products is shown in Figure 5.3. (Figures 5.1, 5.2 and 5.3) highlight the importance of purchased drugs. Street vendors and non-specialized shops come in the second position. This ranking indicates the prevalence of self-medication, while pointing out the financial constraints which are faced by users of healthcare services in the commercial sector.

The reasons for the recourse to self-medication and acquisitions of drugs in non-specialized centers were not explicitly addressed in the current study. However, an analysis of the perception of the households about the cost of

Figure 5.3 Distribution of the households according to the sources of antimalarial drugs

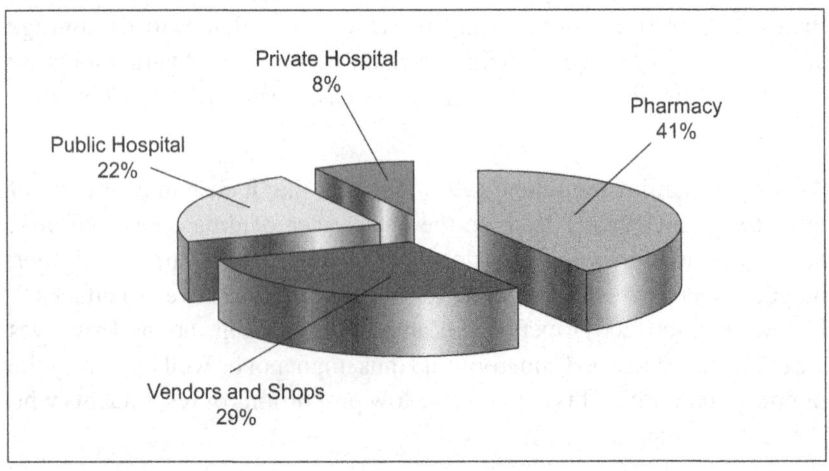

16. Such recommendations are those of the Network for Anti-malaria Therapy created in Yaoundé following a four-day workshop on malaria held in Yaoundé on August 2001 under the supervision of the resident representative of the World Health Organization, Mrs Helen Mambu Madi-Su.

17. As reported in the government newspaper *Cameroon Tribune* of August 20, 2001.

Table 5.6 Distribution of respondents according to known modes of prevention of malaria

Known Prevention Methods	Percentages of Respondents
Does not Know	13.0
Sleep Under a Bed net	45.6
Sleep under an Insecticide-Treated Bed net	5.2
Avoid Mosquito Bites	29.2
Take Preventive Drugs	44.7
Use Traditional Protection Means	1.6
Use insecticide Spirals	7.4
Spraying Insecticides	26.0
Avoid Catching Cold	15.9
Avoid Staying Too Long Under the Sun	5.8
Clean the Surroundings of the Houses	40.0
Drink Clean Water	14.5
Drink Medicinal Tea	1.6
Other	21.1

Notes: The variables are all binary (1 if the respondent mentioned it, 0 otherwise). Hence the percentages can not be summed up along the column.

Source: Compiled by the author based on the survey data.

healthcare indicates that the greatest percentage of the households (32%) think that the drug cost is very high, while 58.3 per cent[18] of the respondents indicated that they had difficulties in securing the funds necessary for their treatment. Moreover, 60.6 per cent of the respondents had to borrow money in order to cover treatment expenses. The annual average cost of healthcare (including transportation, consultation, hospitalization, laboratory expenses, drugs, food and opportunity cost) in the sample was estimated at 48,866 CFA francs, while the median cost was 33,000 CFA francs, and the modal cost was 35,300 CFA francs. When computed on a monthly basis,

18. Based on Ntangsi's analysis (1998), Soula *et al.*, (2000) conclude that 40% of the population in Cameroon may not have the necessary means to cover their basic health needs.

Table 5.7 Distribution of respondents according to modes of malaria prevention practiced

Preventive Methods Practiced	Percentages of Respondents
None	18.7
Sleep Under a Bed net	20.7
Sleep Under an Insecticide-Treated Bed net	1.1
Avoid mosquitoBiites	19.3
Take Preventive Drugs	36.3
Use Traditional Protective Means	2.2
Use Insecticide Spirals	5.9
Spraying Insecticides	24.0
Avoid Catching Cold	10.3
Avoid Staying Too Long Under the Sun	3.4
Clean the Surroundings of the Houses	27.7
Close the Doors and Windows	8.1
Drink Clean Water	12.3
Drink Medicinal Tea	1.4
Other	14.0

Notes: The variables are all binary (1 if the respondent resorted to it, 0 otherwise). Hence the percentages cannot be summed up along the column.

Source: Compiled by the author based on the survey data.

the average cost was 4,075 CFA francs, an amount that is quite comparable to the average expenditure on basic healthcare among poor households determined by (Soula *et al.*, 2000[19]). However, the estimates of treatments expenses for the current study largely exceed those of Ntangsi (1998) that indicate that 5.4 dollars[20] per year for the poorest households but 90.4 dollars per year for the richest.

---

19. The average monthly healthcare expenses are 7,500 cfa francs and 15,000 cfa francs among the poorest and the intermediate households respectively.

20. The current exchange rate of the dollar is 700 CFA Francs for 1 dollar.

5.4.6 Prevention of malaria

Plasmodium falciparum, the principal agent of malaria, has developed a high resistance to chloroquine in Cameroon, the principal drug in the treatment of malaria since 1985, notably in all the bio-climatic zones of the country (Louis, *et al.*, 1994). To deal with such a situation, anti-vectorial control techniques have been developed, with emphasis on the use of chemical products (sprays and anti-mosquito spirals). Hence, it appeared necessary to assess the behavior of the households as far as the preventive methods against malaria were concerned, as well as their attitudes towards the use of bed nets, especially the insecticide-treated ones.

Attitudes towards preventive methods: As shown in table 5.6, the preventive method that is most commonly known to the respondents is the use of untreated bed nets (45.6%). Insecticide-treated bed nets are known by 5.2 per cent of the respondents. About forty five per cent of the respondents think that malaria should be prevented; unfortunately, they did not indicate the type of drug to be taken for that purpose. They probably had in mind a sort of vaccine against malaria. Indeed, the vaccine, SPE66, was tested with muted results in Tanzania: some thirty one per cent protection was obtained after administering the required dose to fifty eight children of one to five years old (Chinmoun, 1997). While a significant percentage of the respondents (40%) know that one can avoid malaria by cleaning the surroundings of the houses, only twenty nine per cent indicated that it is necessary to avoid mosquito bites.

Not only do the respondents know what should be done to prevent malaria, (Table 5.6) but they also resort to various preventive methods against malaria, as indicated in table 5.7. Spraying of insecticides was a common preventive measure undertaken by households. Although the largest proportion of respondents indicated use of preventive drugs, prevention was frequently articulated on the anti-vectorial fight, as evidenced by practices such as bed nets, spraying, clearing the surroundings of the houses, closing windows and doors.

Recourse to the anti-vectoral control: The anti-vectorial control constitutes a significant component of the Cameroonian strategy of malaria control. It is based on the use of the chemical processes (sprays and insecticide spirals). Unfortunately, those practices tend to be too costly, which constitutes a financial burden on the households (Goff *et al.*, 1994). It thus appeared necessary to consider other strategies, which present a better cost-effectiveness ratio for the communities such as the insecticide-treated bed nets.

Most often, people forget that the prevention of malaria starts with the avoidance of the bites of the vector. Yet, the use of bed nets has been known for a long time. Sir R. Ross (1911) advised the use of bed nets at the beginning of the 20th century as an effective measure against malaria. This mode of protection might appear obsolete today but bed nets received a renewed interest thanks to their increased effectiveness upon their impregnation with insecticide of the pyrethrinoid type. The use of insecticide-treated bed nets seems to be an effective solution nowadays in the fight against malaria. Indeed, studies done on a number of countries proved that the use of insecticide-treated bed nets constitutes a promising means for malaria control (Carnavale, Robert, Gazin *et al.*, 1988).

Knowledge and use of insecticide-treated bed nets: Only 5.2 per cent of the respondents (Table 5.6) said that the insecticide-treated bed net is an appropriate means for fighting malaria. In fact, only three out of ten people (29.8%) had heard about insecticide-treated bed nets. Among those, 65.8 per cent did not know where the net could be bought and/or how to get an insecticide-treated bed net. The ministry of public health is the principal source of insecticide-treated bed nets. About 63.4% of respondents said they received their supply from this source. The retreatment of the bed nets is a practice that was not well known by the respondents. However, those who used the insecticide-treated bed nets were ready to have them reprocessed at an average cost of 1,612 CFA francs.

In general, only 15.2 per cent of the respondents had at least one bed net in their household. Among them, more than two thirds (67%) obtained the nets from the market at less than 10,000 CFA francs. The average cost of an ordinary bed net was estimated at 8,084 CFA francs, while the median cost was 6,000 CFA francs.

It should be noted that the National Program of Malaria Control and the Laboratory of Public Health of the Organization of Coordination for the Fight Against the Endemic Diseases in Central Africa (OCEAC) have established a distribution program of insecticide-treated bed nets in healthcare centers of Yaoundé and Douala. The objective of the program is to promote through healthcare centers, the use of insecticide-treated bed nets in the population, and to train medical personnel in techniques of impregnation of bed nets. In order to assess the effectiveness of the implementation of such a policy, Fondjo *et al.*, (2000) evaluated the acceptability of the bed nets among households in Douala. Their results revealed a great degree of unawareness about the insecticide-treated bed nets. Indeed, they noted that bed nets were being used by about fifty per cent of the households, but the recourse to other preventive methods, such as sprays and insecticide spirals were quite frequent. These cost about 50,000 CFA francs per year, compared to 6,000 CFA francs and 4,000 CFA francs spent on large and small-size bed nets, respectively.

5.4.7 Demand for Malaria Control Products and Services

The determinants of the demand for malaria control products and services were identified based on three separate Probit models defined on the following: (a) drug use (which equals 1 if a given drug was being used and equal to 0 otherwise, (b) drug source (which equals 1 for a modern facility and 0 for street vendors); and (c) provision of malaria services (which equals 1 if any hospital service was used and 0 for self-medication). Out of 400 respondents, 170 to 190 provided answers to all the questions related to the variables included in the estimated models. Probit estimation results are shown in tables 5.8, 5.9 and 5.10.

Drug use

Two of the most commonly used drugs, quinine and chloroquine, are analyzed in terms of the probability of their usage. As shown in table 5.8, the probability that an individual would use chloroquine is the least sensitive to the selected variables. Only four out of the twenty-four explanatory variables included in the model significantly affect the probability of using chloroquine. In contrast, eight of these variables significantly affect the probability of using quinine.

The effects of the characteristics of drugs

Prices of drugs: In the two cases analyzed, the law of demand is verified: the price effect on demand is negative and significant in both chloroquine

Table 5.8 A probit model for the use of anti-malaria drugs

Dependent variable: Drug use (equals 1 if a particular drug is being used and 0 for other types of drugs)

Variables	**Coefficients**	
	Chloroquine	**Quinine**
Constant	14.3990 (1.50)	-2.3199 (-0.39)
Drug Prices: Price of Anti-pyretic Drugs	0.6471 (1.29)	0.8916 (2.26)
Price of Chloroquine	-3.3911 (-2.74)	1.3101 (2.16)
Price of Quinine	0.9883 (1.19)	-2.0907 (-3.51)
Price of Other Anti-malaria	-0.0784 (-0.17)	0.2592 (0.84)
Drug acquiring facility (1 = modern)	-0.1560 (-0.46)	–
Source of Service (1 = modern facility)	–	0.2576 (1.11)
Individual level		
Laborer	-0.0931 (-0.27)	-0.1682 (-0.56)
Administrative	-0.1274 (-0.22)	1.2702 (1.98)
Tradesman	-0.1278 (-0.33)	-0.4334 (-1.35)
Agriculture	-1.0710 (-0.71)	1.1570 (1.44)
Education: Primary School	-0.0019 (-0.001)	0.5900 (0.75)
Secondary O-level	-0.3005 (-0.33)	1.1026 (1.38)
Secondary A-level	0.1018 (0.11)	1.3248 (1.66)
University	-0.1617 (-0.17)	1.1044 (1.32)
Residence: Urban Commercial	-0.2147 (-0.39)	0.9088 (1.75)
Urban Popular	-0.2855 (-0.78)	0.3542 (1.05)
Rural	0.5386 (0.58)	0.4821 (0.42)
Religion: Christian	-1.0959 (-1.61))	0.0945 (0.14)
Muslim	-0.7866 (-1.08)	0.4116 (0.56)
Sex (1 = male)	0.5541 (1.85)	0.4354 (1.69)
Age	0.0032 (0.22)	-0.0316 (-2.34)
Number of Malaria Attacks	-0.663 (-0.96)	-0.0305 (-0.55)

Continued

Table 5.8 *(continued)*

Variables	Coefficients	
	Chloroquine	**Quinine**
Household level: Young Children	-0.2031 (-1.51)	-0.1137 (-1.06)
Older Children	-0.0337 (-0.48)	0.1149 (1.84)
Number of Malaria Cases	0.1193 (2.16)	-0.0427 (-0.84)
Pseudo R^2	0.2899	0.2597
Number of Observations	175	178

Note: The reference dummies are; unemployed, illiterate, urban upper class and traditional religion, respectively (*t*-statistics in parentheses).

and quinine demand models. The antipyretic drugs are complementary to either chloroquine or quinine as expected. It is rather counterintuitive to have a complementary relationship between chloroquine and quinine, as evidenced by the positive cross-price effects in the two equations. Such a combination of the two drugs is not clinically defined. Yet, in cases of self-medication, a sick person may start by taking one of those drugs and move on to the second one in a given episode of malaria, without the combination being a prescribed one. Finally, other drugs such as amodiaquine, artemisinin, halofandrine and proguanil, are substitutes for either chloroquine or quinine, but the cross-price effect on each is not significant. It should be recalled that although both quinine and chloroquine are the main affordable malaria treatment drugs in Cameroon, they are associated with high risks of resistance. Because of the risk that Plasmodium Falciparum may be resistant to chloroquine and quinine, it may be neccessary to switch to other drugs in complicated cases of malaria. In view of this, there are considerations at the national level to switch to amodiaquine, another less expensive anti-malarial drug.

Effects of facilities: The dummy for the drug source (0 for street vendors and 1 for modern facilities) is specified only for the chloroquine equation. This dummy has a negative effect as expected. Indeed, chloroquine and quinine unlike other anti-malaria drugs, can be easily obtained from the street vendors.

Table 5.9 Probit model for sources of drugs

Dependent variable: Drug source (equals 1 if modern facility and 0 for street vendors)

Variables	Coefficients	Marginal effects
Constant	-25.5873 (-3.67)	–
Drug Prices: Price of Anti-pyretic Drugs	-1.3714 (-2.95)	-0.3559 (-2.89)
Price of Chloroquine	1.5593 (3.21)	0.4047 (2.95)
Price of Quinine	1.4686 (2.59)	0.3812 (2.60)
Price of Other Anti-malaria	-0.8396 (-2.03)	-0.2179 (-1.94)
Types of Drugs: Anti-pyretics	-0.5233 (-1.33)	-0.1358 (-1.35)
Chloroquine	0.3371 (0.75)	0.08751 (0.76)
Quinine	0.5446 (1.49)	0.1413 (1.55)
Other Anti-malaria Drugs	-0.2758 (-0.72)	-0.0716 (-0.73)
Cost of Healthcare	4.2665 (3.52)	1.1073 (3.18)
Cost of Healthcare Squared	-0.2353 (-3.27)	-0.0611 (-3.00)
Source of Service (1 = hospital)	1.3259 (3.38)	0.3441 (3.68)
Individual level: Laborer	0.1203 (0.27)	0.0312 (0.27)
Administrative	0.1543 (0.20)	0.0401 (0.20)
Tradesman	-0.0434 (-0.10)	-0.0113 (-0.10)
Agriculture	3.2914 (2.50)	0.8542 (2.32)
Education: Primary School	0.6779 (0.91)	0.1759 (0.91)
Secondary O-level	1.3441 (1.34)	0.3488 (1.65)
Secondary A-level	0.8288 (1.05)	0.2151 (1.05)
University	1.8975 (1.94)	0.4924 (2.06)
Religion: Christian	-0.9397(-0.86)	-0.2439(-0.87)
Muslim	-1.2604(-1.10)	-0.3271(-1.13)
Sex (1 = male)	-0.3215(-0.82)	-0.0812(-0.85)
Age	-0.0028(-0.16)	-0.0007(-0.16)

Continued

Table 5.9 *(continued)*

Variables	Coefficients	Marginal effects
Household level: Young Children	-0.0197 (-0.18)	-0.0051 (-0.18)
Older Children	0.0740 (0.95)	0.0192 (0.94)
Pseudo R^2 Number of Observations	0.5023170 170	Predicted probability = 0.8231

Note: The reference dummies are; unemployed, illiterate, urban upper class and traditional religion, respectively (*t*-statistics in parentheses).

Source: Compiled by the author.

Effects of service source: Since chloroquine and quinine are easily accessible, one would expect the source of service dummy (0 for self-medication and 1 for hospital service) to negatively and significantly affect chloroquine and quinine intake. However, this dummy has been specified only in the quinine equation where its effect is positive and non-significant. The positive relationship depicted may be due to the fact that quinine has been one of the most prescribed drugs in most African countries.

Individual level variables

Major activity: In the case of quinine intake, the *ceteris paribus* effect of a person holding an administrative position is estimated to be significantly positive; however, the effect is negative and non-significant in the chloroquine equation.

An interesting finding in table 5.9 appears to be the non-significant negative effect of all the dummies for major activity on chloroquine intake. This finding contradicts the fact that chloroquine is the primary affordable anti-malaria drug in the country. We would have expected a positive coefficient on this variable at least for laborers and those having agriculture as a main activity, given that those groups account for the largest number of the poor (Kamgnia and Timnou, 2000) who rely on cheap drugs. The finding may be a reflection of the fact that physicians and patients are shying away from these two drugs due to resistance of Plasmodium falciparum to quinine and chloroquine in complicated cases of malaria. Other notable results include the following:

Effect of education: Being educated might mean being informed about the side effects of drugs, being able to follow the prescribed dosages and being attentive to risks of drug resistance. We would therefore expect negative effects of education dummies on the probability of using quinine or chloroquine. Such effects are verified for chloroquine. Positive effects are obtained mainly for quinine, such effects being significant only for A-level education.

Effects of area of residence: A positive effect on quinine intake is obtained for some urban areas. Such an effect is quite strong in the commercial urban areas. As regards chloroquine use, the effect is positive, but insignificant in rural areas. However, living in either a commercial or a popular area negatively affects the probability of using chloroquine, which is intuitively reasonable: individuals in those areas are generally better off and can afford to use other drugs to avoid the risk of malaria being resistant to chloroquine.

The effect of gender is positive and significant in the two cases. That is, being a male household head positively affects the probability of using either chloroquine or quinine.

The number of malaria attacks experienced by the household head does not have a significant effect on the use of anti-malaria drugs.

The effect of age is significant only in the case of quinine. It appears that the older an individual gets, the smaller is his demand for quinine.

Household level variables

The number of children, irrespective of the age, negatively affects the demand for chloroquine, although this effect is not significant. However, while the number of younger children (0–5 years old) negatively affects the demand for quinine, the number of older children has a positive and significant effect on the demand for quinine.

The number of malaria cases in the household significantly and positively affects the probability of using chloroquine, which is intuitively reasonable, as the number of malaria cases tends to increase the cost of treatments, and thus pushes the individual to resort to cheap drugs.

Facilities from which drugs were acquired

Respondents indicated that they acquire drugs from street vendors, pharmacies, and public hospitals or private hospitals. Without loss of generality, these facilities were grouped into street vendors versus formal facilities (registered pharmacies, private and public hospitals). The results of the fitted Probit model are as presented in table 5.9. In this table, the most interesting demand effects are those associated with drug types and prices, cost of health care, source of service, and education of the patient.

Anti-malarial drug types and prices

As regards drug prices, all demand effects are significant. However, while the price of either anti-pyretic drugs or other anti-malaria drugs contributes negatively to the probability of acquiring drugs at formal facilities, the prices of quinine and chloroquine have a positive effect. The informal sector remains the second cheapest source of drugs and thus attracts a large number of malaria patients, as found by authors such as Commeyras, Remay and Soula (2000). But popular drugs such as quinine and chloroquine are also available at the formal health centers, especially in catholic and other missionary health facilities. Chloroquine and quinine can be easily obtained over the counter at pharmacies.

Cost of health care: Cost of health care bears a non-linear relationship with the probability of acquiring malaria drugs at the formal facilities, as revealed by the negative and significant coefficient of the square of the cost variable. Indeed, only 58.31 per cent of patients indicated that they had problems in financing the cost of their care. One would then expect the probability of obtaining drugs at formal facilities to increase with the cost of health care, to a level beyond which further cost increases would induce individuals resort to informal facilities.

Source of services: The source of service dummy (0 for self-medication and 1 for hospital service) positively and significantly affects the probability of obtaining anti-malaria drugs at the formal facilities, which is intuitively reasonable. Commeyras, Remay and Soula (2000) point out that while poor households tend to resort to self-medication and acquire the bulk of their drugs from street vendors, rich households rely on hospital services.

Education: Overall, education increases the probability of acquiring anti-malarial drugs from formal facilities. More specifically, the higher the level

Table 5.10 Probit model for sources of malaria services

Dependent variable: Provision of malaria services (equals 1 if hospital service is used and 0 for self-medication)

Variables	Coefficients	Marginal effects
Constant	2.6334 (0.80)	–
Economic Variables		
Cost of Healthcare	-0.7724 (-0.97)	-0.3066 (-0.97)
Cost of Healthcare Square	0.0802 (1.62)	0.0318 (1.62)
Individual level: Laborer	-0.3627 (-1.23)	-0.1440 (-1.23)
Administrative	-1.1543 (-2.35)	-0.4582 (-2.34)
Tradesman	-0.6307 (-1.99)	-0.2503 (-1.97)
Agriculture	-0.1727 (-0.24)	-0.0686 (-0.24)
Education: Primary School	-1.8170 (-2.13)	-0.7212 (-2.13)
Secondary O level	-1.6367 (-1.89)	-0.6496 (-1.90)
Secondary A level	-1.7146 (-1.97)	-0.6805 (-1.97)
University	-1.3196 (-1.46)	-0.5237 (-1.46)
Religion: Christian	0.5277 (0.90)	0.2094 (0.90)
Muslim	0.5100 (0.83)	0.2020 (0.83)
Number of Malaria attacks in the Year	0.0162 (0.25)	0.0064 (0.25)
Household level: ***Young Children***	-0.0655 (-0.54)	-0.0260 (-0.54)
Older Children	0.0319 (0.50)	0.0127 (0.50)
Number of Malaria Cases	-0.1593 (-2.68)	-0.0632 (-2.68)
Pseudo R^2 Number of observations	0.2976 169[21]	Predicted probability = 0.5404

Note: The reference dummies are; unemployed, illiterate, urban upper class and traditional religion respectively (*t*-statistics in parentheses).

Source: Compiled by the author.

[21] Out of the 400 respondents, 170 to 190 provided answers to all the questions related to the variables included in the estimated models.

of education, the more likely it is that the individual would purchase drugs at modern facilities. Indeed, being educated allows individuals to assess the risk of obtaining drugs from informal facilities. Although street vendors provide drugs at low cost, the quality of those drugs is often uncertain and their source rather dubious.

Provision of malaria services

It is assumed that the choice of service provider is a function of cost of healthcare, individual attributes (main activity of the household head, education, religion, number of malaria episodes) and household level characteristics (number of children and malaria cases in the household). The estimated Probit model for source of malaria services is as presented in table 5.10.

The main activity as well as education dummies affect negatively and significantly the probability of using hospital services (Table 5.10), and appears rather counterintuitive. Being in administrative position or being a tradesman should have had a positive effect. Indeed, under normal conditions, being a tradesman would mean being wealthy and the effect of the associated dummy would be to increase the probability of seeking hospital services, as pointed out by Commeyras, Remay and Soula (2000). However, given the gloomy economic environment in Cameroon, being either a trader or an administrator is no longer synonymous with being economically better off.

Being educated could as well mean being aware of the side effects of self-medication. However, in the current case, the more educated the individual is, the less likely it is that he would demand hospital services. It might be that the cost effect has outweighed that of the risk of poor service provision. Moreover, education in many African countries does not necessary mean being wealthy. Hence, self-medication in the form of using old prescriptions or following suggestions from relatives or friends or pharmacists appears to be the most likely behavior among educated individuals, especially in the cases of non-complicated malaria episodes. Nevertheless, educated patients resorting to self-medication does not mean that they acquire drugs from the street vendors, as revealed by the drug source model. Indeed, the individual would demand hospital services as the number of malaria episodes increases, as indicated by the positive, though non-significant coefficient on the number of malaria attacks in the estimated model (Table 5.10). It should be recalled that early recourse to hospital implies proper treatment and thus avoidance of drug resistance or more importantly, avoidance of death due to malaria.

Another interesting finding is the coefficient on the number of malaria cases in the household, which is negative and significant. In fact, as the number of malaria cases increases, individuals are expected to lean toward cost effective treatment as a distinct choice over the security that the modern service provider assures.

5.5 Conclusions and Recommendations

As in many other developing countries, malaria constitutes a major public health problem in Cameroon. Not only does it constitute the primary cause of absenteeism from work and the main reason for consultation in healthcare centers, but also Plasmodium falciparum has developed, especially in the areas of the highest malaria endemicity of the country, strong resistance to chloroquine, which is the primary affordable drug in the treatment of malaria. Therefore, the fight against malaria requires the design and implementation of more encompassing strategies, and consequently, knowledge of the characteristics of the disease as well as of behavior of the patients and that of health care givers.

The study dealt with the demand for malaria control products and services in the urban community of Yaoundé. Its specific objectives were: (i) to determine the degree of awareness about malaria and extent of use of drugs, insecticides and bed nets for the treatment and/or the prevention of malaria; and (ii) to identify the socioeconomic factors which determine the demand for drugs, insecticides and bed nets.

A representative sample of 400 households, distributed over the four health districts of the urban community of Yaoundé was selected. Information collected concerned socio-demographic characteristics of households; the state of knowledge about malaria, its modes of transmissions and methods of prevention; the therapeutic behavior, knowledge and use of anti-malarial drugs; knowledge of and use of bed nets, as well as of insecticide-treated bed nets, especially for the protection of children, and pregnant women.

The results of the study indicate that the majority of the respondents knew about malaria, its modes of transmission and its methods of prevention. However, only a few of the respondents knew about the protection provided by insecticide-treated bed nets. As regards therapeutic aspects, self-medication constitutes the main mode of treatment; quinine stands out as the most commonly used product along with the antipyretic drugs, these being acquired primarily from pharmacies.

As for the demand for malaria control products and services, factors determining the probability of using the most popular drugs (chloroquine or quinine) are prices of the drugs, education, sex, age, and number of children. More specifically, the law of demand is verified in those two cases: the own price effect is negative and statistically significant. The antipyretic drugs are complementary to either chloroquine or quinine as expected. Concerning the probability of using hospital services, the determinants of that probability are the cost of healthcare (a significant nonlinear effect was found), the main activity of the household head (significantly negative effects of different categories were detected, which could be due to the then gloomy economic environment), the education of the household head, and the number of malaria cases he had (a negative and significant effect was found).

The facility from which drug was obtained (equals 1 if modern facility and 0 street vendors) happened to be the most important factor in the demand for malaria treatments. The major determinants of the demand for drugs at the formal facilities are the prices of drugs, the cost of health care and education of the patient.

In sum, three points could be made about the results of this study. The first point is that the cost of health care remains a major policy variable in the fight against poverty in general, and against malaria in particular. Given that hospital services for consultation or for malaria control products are unaffordable beyond a certain cost level, such a level needs to be determined to serve as a benchmark in the specification of user fees in Cameroon. However, even though user fees might be necessary, they should be levied at levels that would not drive individuals away from modern health institutions. The second point is that campaigns against malaria, combined with health information, would benefit individuals as well as communities.

The third point is that if households could get well informed, that is, if they were to have access to appropriate health education, they would resort to effective ways of treating malaria. That is, they would not only use the most effective treatment, but also patronize modern facilities which are the cheapest way of controlling malaria in Cameroon.

References

Basco, L. (2001), "Mise au point: Nouveaux medicaments antipaludiques disponibles en Afrique", *Le Bulletin de liaison et de documentation de l'OCEAC,* 2° Trismestre.

Bitchong, E.C. (1997), *Les formes graves du paludisme chez l'enfant à l'hôpital général de Yaoundé : aspects clinique, biologique et évolution,* Thèse de doctorat en Médecine, Université de Yaoundé I.

Carnavale, P., Robert, V., and Gazin, P., *et al.,* (1988), «Influence des moustiquaires imprégnées de delméthrine (à 25 mg/m2) dans la réduction de la transmission du paludisme humain dans un village des environs de Bobo-Dioulasso (Burkina Faso)» Bull. Soc. Path. Ex., 81, 832–846.

Chinmoun, D. (1997), *Etude comparée de l'efficacité et tolérance clinique de l'Artemether et de la Quinine dans le traitement de l'accès pernicieux palustre de l'enfant de 0 à 10 ans à Yaoundé,* Thèse de doctorat en Médecine, Université de Yaoundé I.

Comeyras, C., Remay, S., and Soula, G., (2000), « Problématique du médicament au Cameroun. Etat des lieux de l'offre, de la demande, des prix de vente, et perspectives pour améliorer l'accessibilité financière », *Bulletin doc OCEAC,* Volume 33 (4), p 23–30.

Direction de la Statistique et de la Comptabilité Nationale (1996), *Enquête ECAM. Direction de la statistique et de la comptabilité nationale.* MINEFI, Yaoundé.

Direction de la Statistique et de la Comptabilité Nationale (1998), *Annuaire Statistique du Cameroun,* Direction de la statistique et de la comptabilité nationale. MINEFI, Yaoundé.

Dor, A., Gertler, P. and van der Gaag, J. (1987), "Non-Price Rationing and the Choice of Medical Care Providers in Rural Côte d'Ivoire". *Journal of Health Economics, vol. 6:* 291–304.

Dow, W. (1999), "Flexible Discrete Choice Demand Models Consistent with Utility Maximization: An Application to Health Care Demand". *American Journal of Agricultural Economics, vol 81:* 680–685.

Duchesne, D. (1998), « Evaluation de la fonction de la demande de soins de santé en Tanzanie », Centre de Recherche et de Développement en Economique, Université de Montréal.

Eboh, E., and Okeibunor, J.C. (1998), "Consequences of Malaria Disease on Farm Labor Supply, Labor Productivity and Resource Allocation among Households in Omor Community Anambra State, Nigeria". *les cahiers de l'IFORD*, n° 15, 94 p.

Fambon, S. *et al.*, (2001), *Réformes économiques et pauvreté au Cameroun durant les années 1990,* rapport projet collaboratif sur la pauvreté, CREA.

Fondjo, E., *et al.*, (2000), *Evaluation de l'acceptabilité des moustiquaires imprégnées dans 5 formations sanitaires de la ville de Douala en 1999–2000*, Document Technique, OCEAC N° 1090/LSP. Fotso M. *et al.*, (1999), Enquête Démographique et de Santé du Cameroun (EDSC-II) – 1998. BUCREP/ Macro International Inc. Calverton, Maryland USA.

Gallup, J.L. and Sachs, J.D. (2000), *Economics of Malaria.* Harvard School of Public Health.

Gbary, A. R.(1999), *Revue de «Faire Reculer le Paludisme en Afrique,* Réunion de consensus, de planification pour l'évaluation des besoins et développement des stratégies de l'initiative « Faire Reculer le Paludisme en Afrique », Yaoundé, 26–29 avril 1999.

Gourieroux, C. (1989), Économétrie des Variables Qualitatives, 2ème Edition, Economica.

Greene, H.W. (2000), *Econometric Analysis*. Fourth Edition, Prentice Hall.

Juillet, A. (1999), « L'Impact des tarifs des services de santé et des revenus sur les décisions de recours aux soins des malades à Bamako », *Revue d'Economie du Développement*, n°4, Décembre.

Kamgnia, D.B., and Timnou, J.P. (2001), Pauvreté au Cameroun : Evolution dans une conjoncture d'ajustement économique, Rapport final, projet CREA.

Kassankogno, Y. (1999a), *Le partenariat global « Faire Reculer le Paludisme » : une introduction.* Réunion de consensus, de planification pour l'évaluation des besoins et développement des stratégies de l'initiative « Faire Reculer le Paludisme en Afrique », Yaoundé, 26–29 avril 1999.

Kassankogno, Y. (1999b), *Etat et expérience dans la mise en œuvre du programme accéléré de lutte contre le paludisme*, Réunion de consensus, de planification pour l'évaluation des besoins et développement des stratégies de l'initiative « Faire Reculer le Paludisme en Afrique », Yaoundé, 26–29 avril 1999.

Magda, R. (1999), *Les interventions techniques disponibles et la base de leur sélection*, Réunion de consensus, de planification pour l'évaluation des besoins et développement des stratégies de l'initiative « Faire Reculer le Paludisme en Afrique », Yaoundé, 26–29 avril 1999.

Miller, I. and Freund, J.E. (1985), *Probability and Statistics for Engineers*. Third Edition, Prentice-Hall.

Ministère de la Santé Publique, Cameroun (1999), *Carte Sanitaire du Cameroun. Ministère de la santé publique,* Yaoundé, juin 1999.

Ministère de la Santé Publique, Cameroun (2000b), *Analyse situationnelle du paludisme au niveau national*, Rapport d'analyse (draft), Ministère de la santé publique, Yaoundé, août 2000.

Ministère de la Santé Publique, Cameroun (2001), *Plan d'action de lutte contre le paludisme au Cameroun biennium 2000–200,* Ministère de la santé publique, Yaoundé, janvier 2001.

Ministère de la Santé Publique, Cameroun (2.000a), *Stratégie Sectorielle de Santé,* Plan National du Développement Sanitaire, Yaoundé, Juin 2000.

Nájera, J.A. e*t al.*, (1992), *Malaria: New Patterns and Perspectives*. World Bank Technical Paper No. 183:35.

Ntangsi, J. (1998), "An Analysis of Health Sector Expenditure in Cameroon Using a National Health Accounts Framework", World Bank Resident Mission in Cameroon.

Ross, R (1911), *The Prevention of Malaria:* 2nd edition. London: John Murray.

Sahn, E.D., Younger, D.S., and Genicot, G. (2002), "The Demand for Health Care Services in Rural Tanzania" Cornell University.

Snow, R.W, Rowan, K.M., and Greenwood, B.M. (1987), A Trial of Permethrin Treated Bed Nets in the Prevention of Malaria in Gambian Children, *Trans. Roy. Soc. Trop. Med. Hyg.*, 81, 4, 563–576.

Verbeek, M. (2000), *A Guide to Modern Econometrics*. John Wiley & Sons.

Chapter 5 Appendix Tables

Table 5.A1 Group I: Antipyretic drugs

Source	Paracetamol	Aspirin	Anti-inflamatory
Pharmacy 1	955	705	1,710
Pharmacy 2	845	750	–
Pharmacy 3	1,025	1,215	2,220
Pharmacy 4	730	–	–
Pharmacy 5	1,365	1,215	–
Pharmacy 6	–	–	–
Pharmacy 7	500	250	750
Mean	**903,333**	**827**	**1,560**
Variance	**85,346.667**	**163,707.5**	**557,100**
Standard error	**292.14**	**94,206.11**	**746.39**

Table 5.A2 Group II: Amodiaquine

Source	Métamizol	Camoquin 200mg	Camoquin 125mg	Amodia-quine	Flavo-quine
Pharmacy 1	–	2,325	1,990	**1,560**	2,065
Pharmacy 2	–	–	–	**1,625**	3,810
Pharmacy 3	–	–	1,985	**1,560**	2,265
Pharmacy 4	790	–	–	–	–
Pharmacy 5	–	1,260	–	–	2,020
Pharmacy 6	1,550	1,260	1,985	**1,560**	2,265
Pharmacy 7	–	1275	2,000	**1,575**	2,275
Mean	**1,170**	**1,530**	**1,990**	**1,576**	**2,450**
Variance	**1,170**	**280,950**	**50**	**7,92.5**	**456,360**
Standard error	**537.40**	**530.05**	**7.07**	**28.15**	**675.54**

Table 5.A3 Group III: Artemisinin

Source	Arsumax 50mgB/12	Plamotrin 200mg B/6	Paluther 40mg inj	Paluther 80mg inj	Arinate	Arteme-ther	Cotexcim
Pharmacy 1	3,820	4,245	7,235	12,520	3,178	–	3,680
Pharmacy 2	4,275	7,195	–	–	3,150	–	3,680
Pharmacy 3	3,810	–	–	–	–	–	–
Pharmacy 4	3,810	4,225	6,000	–	3,125	5,220	3,680
Pharmacy 5	3,210	4,225	–	–	3,225	–	3,680
Pharmacy 6	3,810	4,225	7,195	12,490	3,125	5,220	3,665
Pharmacy 7	3,825	4,225	7,250	12,525	3,105	–	3,665
Mean	**3,794.28**	**4,723.33**	**6,920**	**12,511.67**	**3,151.33**	**5,220**	**3,675**
Variance	**95,803.57**	**1,466,256.67**	**63,586,764.67**	**358.333**	**1,934.67**	**0**	**60**
Standard error	**309.52**	**1,210.89**	**7,974.13**	**18.93**	**43.98**	**0**	**7.746**

Table 5.A4 Group IV: Chloroquine

Source	Nivaquine 100mg	Nivaquine 300mg	Nivaquine/ Chloroquin	Melubrin 250mg	Melubrin SP	Risochin 100mg	Risochin 250mg	Aralen 300mg
Pharmacy 1	1,170	1,550	**2,195**	710	1,650	2,020	2,670	620
Pharmacy 2	180	1,980	**1,810**	–	1,375	–	2,675	–
Pharmacy 3	1,170	1,435	**1,800**	–	–	–	–	–
Pharmacy 4	–	–	–	–	–	–	–	–
Pharmacy 5	1,000	–	–	–	–	–	–	–
Pharmacy 6	2,925	1,500	**2,195**	1,640	–	2,670	–	–
Pharmacy 7	950	1,485	**1,625**	1,635	1,650	2,025	2,675	–
Mean	**1,232.5**	**1,590**	**1,925**	**1,328.33**	**1,558.33**	**2,238.33**	**2,673.33**	**620**
Variance	**822,797.5**	**49,212.5**	**66,162.5**	**286,758.33**	**25,208.33**	**139,758.33**	**8.33**	**0**
Standard error	**907.08**	**221.84**	**257.22**	**535.50**	**158.77**	**373.84**	**2.89**	**0**

Table 5.A5 Group V: Cycline

Source	Doxycyclines 100mg	Tetracycline
Pharmacy 1	937	1,165
Pharmacy 2	1,855	1,170
Pharmacy 3	–	1,165
Pharmacy 4	–	1,170
Pharmacy 5	1,000	1,165
Pharmacy 6	–	–
Pharmacy 7	1,000	1,175
Mean	**1,198**	**1,168.333**
Variance	**192,726**	**16.667**
Standard error	**439.01**	**4.08**

Table 5.A6 Group VI: Halofantrine

Source	Halphan Cp	Halphan SP
Pharmacy 1	5,390	4,030
Pharmacy 2	5,370	4,010
Pharmacy 3	5,390	4,030
Pharmacy 4	–	–
Pharmacy 5	5,390	–
Pharmacy 6	5,390	4,030
Pharmacy 7	5,400	4,900
Mean	**5,388.33**	**4,200**
Variance	**96.67**	**153,200**
Standard error	**9.83**	**391.41**

Table 5.A7 Group VII : Lumefantrine+artemisinin

Source	Coartem P/8	Coartem P/16
Pharmacy 1	2,980	4,975
Pharmacy 2	2,980	4,950
Pharmacy 3	–	4,985
Pharmacy 4	–	–
Pharmacy 5	4,995	–
Pharmacy 6	2,980	–
Pharmacy 7	3,000	4,975
Mean	**3,322.5**	**4,971.25**
Variance	**808,095**	**222.92**
Standard error	**898.94**	**14.93**

Table 5.A8 Group VIII : Proguanil

Source	Paludrine
Pharmacy 1	6,515
Pharmacy 2	6,515
Pharmacy 3	–
Pharmacy 4	6,530
Pharmacy 5	6,530
Pharmacy 6	6,530
Pharmacy 7	6,525
Mean	**6,524.17**
Variance	**54.17**
Standard error	**7.38**

Table 5.A9 Group IX: Proguanil+chloroquine

Source	Savarine
Pharmacy 1	8,525
Pharmacy 2	8,525
Pharmacy 3	–
Pharmacy 4	8,040
Pharmacy 5	–
Pharmacy 6	8,540
Pharmacy 7	8,525
Mean	**8,431**
Variance	**47,817.5**
Standard error	**218.672**

Table 5.A10 Group X: Pyrimethamine

Source	Malocide	Daraprim
Pharmacy 1	7,337	2,089
Pharmacy 2	–	2,050
Pharmacy 3	–	2,050
Pharmacy 4	–	2,050
Pharmacy 5	–	2,050
Pharmacy 6	5,700	2,050
Pharmacy 7	–	2,050
Mean	**6,518.5**	**2,055.57**
Variance	**1,339,884.5**	**217.286**
Standard error	**1157.53**	**14.74**

Table 5.A11 Group XI : Pyrimethamine+sulfadoxine

Source	Fansidar CP 500mg	Fansidar 5 00mg inj	Maloxine	Malastop
Pharmacy 1	1,190	2,375	650	580
Pharmacy 2	1,190	–	550	450
Pharmacy 3	1,190	2,325	600	–
Pharmacy 4	1,090	–	650	600
Pharmacy 5	1,190	–	900	600
Pharmacy 6	1,190	2,370	600	475
Pharmacy 7	1,190	2,375	725	450
Mean	**1,175.71**	**2,361.25**	**667.86**	**525.83**
Variance	**1,428.571**	**589.583**	**13,482.143**	**5,604.17**
Standard error	**37.80**	**24.28**	**116.11**	**74.86**

Table 5.A12 Group XII: Pyrimethamine+sulfadoxine+méfloquine

Source	Fansinef
Pharmacy 1	3,765
Pharmacy 2	3,765
Pharmacy 3	3,775
Pharmacy 4	3,770
Pharmacy 5	3,765
Pharmacy 6	3,765
Pharmacy 7	3,765
Mean	**3,767.14**
Variance	**15.47**
Standard error	**3.93**

Table 5.A13 Group XIII : Quinine

Source	Quinoforme	Quinimax	Quinine	Arsiquino-forme
Pharmacy 1	1,775	5,035	**1,805**	3,355
Pharmacy 2	–	–	**1,950**	–
Pharmacy 3	5,030	–	–	3,255
Pharmacy 4	–	–	**1,000**	–
Pharmacy 5	–	5,055	**1,500**	3,210
Pharmacy 6	–	5,055	–	3,210
Pharmacy 7	–	3,225	**2,000**	3,225
Mean	**3,402.5**	**4,592.5**	**1,651**	**3,251**
Variance	**5,297,512.5**	**1,104,233.3**	**170,380**	**3,717.5**
Standard error	**2,301.63**	**911.72**	**412.77**	**60.97**

Source: Survey data.

Chapter 6

The Distribution of Pharmaceutical Products and Malaria Control in Zambia

Flora M. Musonda, Francis Mangani

6.0 Introduction

Malaria is a serious disease caused by a parasite called plasmodium. The malaria parasite spends part of its life cycle in a mosquito and the other one in a human being. There are four types of plasmodium parasites that are known to cause malaria in human beings. These are *plasmodium falciparum, plasmodium malariae, plasmodium vivax* and *plasmodium ovale.* These parasites survive by feeding on blood. It is through this process of feeding that the plasmodium is transmitted from one human being to the other. When a mosquito bites someone who is infected, it sucks blood containing the plasmodium that causes malaria. And when the same mosquito bites another person who is not infected it injects the malaria parasite into that person.

In human beings, when the plasmodium is injected into the blood stream, it attacks the liver where maturation and multiplication occur. From the liver, the parasites enter the red blood cells. In these cells, the parasites further mature and multiply until the cells burst (hemolysis). This releases the mature parasites and toxic materials into the blood stream where they move and enter the liver cells again and the process is repeated. During the time the parasites are in the liver the person may feel fever, nausea and vomiting, headache, abdominal pains and general body pains. Sometimes these parasites can invade organs such as the brain and cause cerebral malaria or the kidneys and cause black water fever. These could be severe forms of malaria and can cause death.

6.1 Malaria in Zambia

In Zambia, plasmodia that cause severe forms of malaria exist. Although there are four categories identified, these plasmodia differ significantly in how much they account for malaria cases in different geographical regions. In Zambia today, plasmodia can be split into the following categories:

- Plasmodium falciparum, which accounts for ninety five per cent of all malaria cases in Zambia;
- Plasmodium malariae, account for five per cent of the malaria cases;
- Plasmodium ovale, account for two per cent of malaria cases; and
- Plasmodium vivax, is very rare in Zambia and its effect very insignificant.

By about 1985, the government of Zambia had successfully driven the major vector (i.e. the mosquito) from most of the urban habitats. With the abundant resources at that time, the government was able to combat malaria through its residue household spraying campaign in urban areas, though not much was done in rural areas.

In Zambia, malaria is the leading cause of ill health and death. It accounts for about twenty four per cent of all health center admissions and twelve per cent of hospital admissions. Statistics indicate that between twelve per cent and twenty per cent of deaths are due to malaria. Table 6.1 shows the trend in malaria as a proportion of hospital morbidity and death. The table shows that there was an increase in the number of admissions for malaria from 1976 to 1994.

It must be mentioned here that these figures are recorded at facility level. The implication of this is that these are rough estimates of the true picture of the malaria situation in Zambia. Some malaria cases are not reported at the facility level. Malaria is now an endemic disease in Zambia with North Western Province being the most affected at 590 cases per 1000, followed by Luapula Province at 490 cases per 1000. Lusaka's incidence is estimated at 265 cases per 1000 (NMCC, 2000). Generally, the incidence of malaria has continued to increase exponentially, and the most affected are children under five years and pregnant women.

Table 6.1 Malaria morbidity in Zambia, 1976–1994

Year	Total Health Center and Hospital Outpatient Morbidity for Malaria	Malaria as a Proportion of Total HC and Hospital Outpatient	Total Hospital Admission for Malaria	Malaria as a Proportion of Total Hospital Admissions
1976	590,681	–	36,057	8.8
1977	627,561	–	42,375	10.1
1978	713,739	–	48,418	11.5
1979	761,636	–	46,096	10.9
1980	877,360	–	51,054	11.4
1981	972,285	–	49,374	10.6
1982	1,008,094	–	61,432	12.2
1983	1,287,621	–	81,739	14.4
1984	1,451,396	–	91,848	16.7
1985	1,557,267	10.2	92,641	16.8
1986	1,515,410	10.5	103,238	17.7
1987	1,530,733	–	–	–
1988	2,158,343	–	–	–
1989	1,055,473	8.1	107,270	21.9
1990	1,933,013	16.8	126,912	22
1991	2,153,149	20.6	119,109	20.6
1992	2,957,308	21.0	113,378	19.6
1993	–	–	132,745	–
1994	72,516	–	112,569	–

Source: Bulletins of Health Statistics, Major Health Trends, Ministry of Health, 1976–1998.

Table 6.2 shows the Malaria Incidence Rates from 1976 to 1998 as diagnosed by the public health system while table 6.3 shows the Malaria Incidence Rates per 1000 Population, nationally and by province, 1996 and 1997.

Table 6.2 shows that between 1976 and 1986, there was an increase of 924,729 in the number of malaria cases. This shows a percentage increase

Table 6.2 Malaria incidence rates from 1976 to 1998 in Zambia

Year	Total Estimated Population	No. of New Malaria Cases	Incidence Rate/ 1000
1976	4,859,860	590,681	122
1977	5,029,955	627,561	125
1978	5,206,003	713,739	137
1979	5,388,213	761,636	141
1980	5,576,801	877,360	157
1981	5,837,317	972,285	167
1982	6,018,274	1,008,094	168
1983	6,204,840	1,287,621	208
1984	6,397,190	1,451,396	227
1985	6,725,300	1,557,267	232
1986	6,967,819	1,515,410	218
1987	7,228,056	1,530,733	212
1988	7,496,997	2,158,343	288
1989	7,565,769	1,993,262	260
1990	7,818,447	1,993,696	247
1991	8,080,682	2,340,994	290
1992	8,352,848	2,953,629	354
1993	8,457,523	3,514,000	416
1994	8,764,180	2,742,188	313
1995	–	–	355
1996	–	–	378
1997	9,640,122	–	383
1998	9,910,035	–	399

Source: Bulletins of Health Statistics, Major Health Trends, Ministry of Health, 1976–1998.

of 157 per cent from 1986 onward, the trend does not seem to differ significantly from the previous one.

From table 6.3, it is clear that North Western Province was the hardest hit at 588.8 per 1000 in 1996 and 631.8 per 1000 in 1997 followed by Luapula Province at 484 per 1000 and 519.3 per 1000 in the respective years. Those that are least hit include Lusaka and Southern Provinces with incidence rates of 265.3 and 290 respectively in 1996 and 284.7 and 311.2 in 1997.

Table 6.3 Malaria incidence rates per 1000 population, nationally and by Province

Province	Total Population		Incidence Rate per 1000	
	1996	1997	1996	1997
Central	938,924	965,214	336	360.6
Copperbelt	1,831,448	1,882,728	321	344.2
Eastern	1,248,599	1,283,560	386	414.6
Luapula	604,701	621,633	484	519.3
Lusaka	1,692,741	1,740,138	265	284.7
Northern	1,008,180	1,036,409	326	350
North-Western	446,779	459,289	589	631.8
Southern	1,167,853	1,200,552	290	311.2
Western	700,887	720,511	442	474.5
National	9,640,112	9,910,035	383	398.8

Source: Bulletins of Health Statistics, Major Health Trends, Ministry of Health, 1976–1998.

Over the period from 1986 to 1996, malaria incidence increased from 122 to 360 cases per 1000, a three-fold increase. Unfortunately, all this happened even though malaria is not only treatable but is also a preventable disease. Goodman *et al.*, (2000), identified the following as key preventive measures against malaria:

- Use of insecticide treated nets;
- Chemoprophylaxis for children;
- Residue Spraying;

- Chemoprophylaxis in pregnancy;
- Potential malaria vaccines;
- Other prevention interventions.

Because of its high levels of prevalence, malaria has become a serious menace to economic and social development throughout the world and Sub-Saharan Africa is no exception. It is exerting a very significant negative impact on the overall national development.

Malaria has become a threat to health and development because the government currently lacks sufficient resources to run anti-malaria campaigns as in the past. In addition to the government's inadequacy of resources, the financial and material support that used to come from the copper mines is no longer there, except from a few companies such as Konkola Copper Mines, which have launched an anti-malaria campaign in Chingola and Chililabombwe (WHO, 2001), and the Mopani Copper Mines in Kitwe and Mufulira. The mines and mining companies have played a significant role in the fight against malaria in the past. Due to the lack of resources in all health fronts, malaria cases have increased markedly over the last twenty years in the country, with the mining towns being no exception. Overall, malaria cases in the Copperbelt increased from about seventy per 1000 in 1970 to about 158 per 1000 in the year 2000. The extent of this increase has been exacerbated by the general increase in poverty in the population.

Malaria has also won the support of the parasite, which in most cases has built up resistance to most of the conventional chemotherapy (NMCC, 2000). The malaria-causing mosquito has in the recent past become increasingly resistant to insecticides, thereby rendering the anti-malaria efforts ineffective. Furthermore, the malaria parasite itself has developed resistance to chloroquine, which is the commonest and most affordable anti-malarial drug in the country.

As the malaria incidence rates get higher, and as the malaria parasites get resistant to the conventional chemotherapy, the cost of treating malaria cases increases as well. This scenario can have serious socioeconomic implications. In Zambia, the malaria prevalence has culminated into the following situations:

- Loss of productivity in the workplace and fields;
- Reductions in potential income and food supply;
- Attention deficits among children and loss of schooling opportunities;
- High funeral and burial expenses;
- High costs of curative care.

6.2 Distribution of Anti-malarial Drugs

There are two major providers of drugs in Zambia, which can be classified as primary and secondary sources. The primary source essentially comprises the local and foreign drug manufacturing and distributing companies; it is hoped that the local firms will dominate the market. The secondary sources comprise non-manufacturing companies, which obtain pharmaceuticals from manufacturing firms and distribute them on behalf of the firms or independently.

Although very few indigenous primary sources of drugs exist in Zambia, the National Drug Policy (NDP) encourages local production through local pharmaceutical companies. In 1991, there were a total of seven pharmaceutical manufacturers who mostly produced generic drugs. Of these seven, three have since closed down due to operational problems and one has been privatized, vis. the Medical Stores Ltd.

A large share of the drug market in Zambia is in the hands of the secondary-source providers, typically, the drug importers. They include multilateral and bilateral donors, Medical Stores Ltd., Ministry of Health, the State House, private firms, NGOs, Christian Medical Association of Zambia (CMAZ), private retail pharmacies, private clinics (including mission health facilities), and individuals who import drugs on a very small scale.

Many importers act as wholesalers, distributing pharmaceutical products directly to health facilities and retail pharmacies. At the end of 1995, there were a total of forty importers and wholesalers in Zambia (Government of Zambia, 1996). However, Zambia Revenue Authority statistics showed that there were more than eighty different organizations, companies, clinics and government bodies involved in the importation of drugs. The Ministry of Health was a major importer, which in monetary terms accounted for about forty six per cent of all drug imports, followed by private importers and donors with shares of thirty per cent and nineteen per cent respectively. Table 6.4 shows the main importers of drugs in Zambia as of 1996.

Wholesaler firms provide drugs at a profit to commercial pharmacies even though at times they sell drugs directly to individual health facilities. The Medical Stores Ltd., which has a somewhat special role in the arena of pharmaceutical drugs, is an example of an organization that imports and distributes drugs directly to the retailers. The Medical Stores Ltd acts mainly as the government's storage and distribution agent, and is responsible for distributing to individual health institutions and districts, the drugs procured directly by Ministry of Health. Medical Stores Ltd. also distributes essential drug kits financed by donors to all health centers, and charges ten per cent of the value of each consignment as the service fee.

Table 6.4 Drug imports (thousands of US dollars), 1996

Importer	Value of Imports	% of Total
Ministry of Health	4,787	45.7%
Other Government Bodies	65	0.6%
Medical Stores Ltd.	297	2.8%
Donors	2,030	19.4%
Private Importers	3,177	30.3%
Mission	62	0.6%
NGOs	59	0.6%
Total	10,477	100%

Source: Societe General De Surveillance (1996).

Pharmaceutical products are mostly provided by health institutions, which encompass government, private outlets such as the mines, private clinics and hospitals and local retailers. The latter are concentrated along the railway line. In Zambia, as in other low-income countries, drugs can be purchased from informal markets including street vendors and drug peddlers.

In the case of government health institutions, drugs are procured by the Ministry of Health. The Government orders drugs from international and local suppliers for delivery to the health ministry, which in turn delivers to respective public health facilities around the country. All local retail pharmacies must register with the Pharmacy and Poisons Board of Zambia to get the drugs.

The first line anti-malarial drug in Zambia is chloroquine (CQ). This has been a drug of choice for the first line treatment of uncomplicated malaria since the beginning of the malaria control efforts, because of its rapid action, efficacy, safety and low cost. CQ is distributed through public health facilities and retail outlets. Nonetheless, there are other anti-malarial drugs that are used to treat malaria, including: fansidar, which is dispensed by health centers and also sold at retail outlets; quinine, which is used particularly for in-patient care; artemesinin drugs; halfantin; and other drugs distributed through the private health care system.

To ensure the prompt, safe and efficient distribution of drugs from the central storage facilities to the entire country, the Government promised to affect the following:

- Establish a reliable and transparent procurement system which shall support the national health care packages through the procurement of generic products at competitive prices;
- Decentralize the procurement process;
- Establish an independent, autonomous, professional and accountable body to ensure the availability of essential drugs using the Zambia National Tender Board regulations;
- Restructure and commercialize the Medical Stores Limited.

At the health center and hospital levels, the drugs for public health facilities are distributed through districts. The districts make requests and the drugs are purchased centrally by the Medical Stores Ltd. The drugs that are purchased by the Medical Stores are pre-packed before delivery. The pre-packed drugs are delivered to various health facilities in packets known as the "essential drug kits," with each packet containing prescribed types and quantities of drugs. In addition to the essential drug kits, there are special drug kits requested by health centers and sent to districts for community health workers.

At the community level, a community health worker, who is normally a trained volunteer, may be allowed to dispense the basic drugs in the special kits to the sick. The community health workers are charged with the task of health promotion, prevention, case detection and case management in their communities. To verify if the drugs bought by Medical Stores are safe to use, all drugs go through a laboratory facility for quality control and physical checking. Table 6.5 shows the value of drugs distributed to hospitals and health centers in the various provinces.

Table 6.5 Value of drugs (US dollars) by province, 1999-2001

Province	1999	2000	2001
Central	69,262,694	6,061,341	22,301.6
Copperbelt	97,002,967	6,511,854	58,533.1
Eastern	88,010,741	21,827,639	20,859.8
Luapula	28,248,743	8,454,486	11,715.5
Lusaka	77,148,557	5,212,517	52,699.2
Northern	65,690,666	16,675,325	15,592.7
North-Western	42,422,473	5,793,161	16,989.0
Southern	102,000,000	11,730,952	27,175.9
Western	36,814,703	13,288,465	13,758.8

Source: Accounting records, Medical Stores Ltd.

Table 6.5 reveals that from 1999 to 2001, the provinces received varying amounts of pharmaceutical drug support, but with a general decline in the amounts received being registered in all provinces. For instance, the Southern Province, which received the largest amount of support with drugs valued at about US$ 102 million in 1999, received drugs valued at only US $ 27,175 in 2001. On the other hand, other provinces like Lusaka and the Copperbelt maintained a proportionately larger amount of support from 1999 to 2001.

Considering that tables 6.3 and 6.5 covered different time periods, it is not possible to draw out perfect comparisons based on the data presented. However, because the data on malaria incidence by province (Table 6.3) were obtained from a time period preceding that of the distribution of drugs by province (Table 6.5), some useful inferences can be made. A surprising observation with regard to the distribution patterns of drugs among the provinces is that the drugs are seen to be distributed in quite a contradictory manner when account is taken of the incidence of malaria in the provinces in the preceding periods. For example, North-Western Province was the hardest hit by malaria in 1996 and 1997, and as such one would expect a larger amount of pharmaceutical support to this region over the period, 1998 to 2001. However, quite the contrary was observed. Provinces such as Lusaka and Southern, which had relatively lower malaria incidences during 1996 and 1997, received proportionately more pharmaceutical support over the same period. Clearly, there is a targeting problem with respect to the distribution of drugs in Zambia.

6.3 The Fight Against Malaria

At independence, Zambia inherited a malaria control program that had urban and rural components, though not surprisingly, the control effort was concentrated in urban areas. There were few health facilities so that access to malaria treatment was poor. After independence, the government increased its health budget and improved health infrastructure. There was a new emphasis on health for all. This was not only an effort to fight malaria alone but other diseases were targeted for control as well.

The Zambian government showed a high level of commitment to improving health at independence in 1964. At the time, concrete measures were taken to improve equity of access to quality care through rapid expansion of the health infrastructure. Whenever economic situation has allowed, the Zambian government has since shown willingness to reform the sector and try new ways of improving health services. Innovation has been a central theme in successive health-sector reform efforts in Zambia.

Unfortunately, however, a poor national economic climate continues to impact negatively on this progress. Both poor growth and currency depreciation have led to a perceptible short fall in the actual resources available for health investments. As a result, in spite of the reforms, there have been significant rises in both morbidity and mortality from malaria. Nationwide, malaria is assuming an increasingly alarming proportion of morbidity and mortality from all causes.

As early as 1932, some pieces of legislation were passed regarding malaria prevention and control. Some of the most notable ones included Mosquito Extermination Act of 1944 which has since been amended several times, the latest being in 1964; and the Mosquito Extermination Act, CAP 537 of 1964. This piece of legislation primarily focussed on keeping villages clean and tidy, as well as ensuring adequate in-door residue spraying with Dichloro-Diphenyl-Trichloroethane (DDT) (0.2g/m^2).

Three independent authorities administered the residue spraying program: the municipal councils were responsible for urban areas, the health ministry was responsible for rural areas, and the mining companies and their contractors were responsible for the mine compounds, with costs in mines being borne by the mining companies alone. Municipal councils shared half of the urban costs with the Ministry of Health.

The residue spraying and household sanitation program was a success because it managed to bring the incidence rates of malaria to a minimum. The focus on the development of urban areas helped to reduce the malaria transmission in urban areas for at least three decades, from 1940–1970. During this period the disease was almost eliminated from the eight principal towns along the line of rail (National Malaria Control Center, 1990).

Today malaria is a serious problem in rural areas. Rural malaria prevention control measures were generally restricted to curative services. Chemoprophylaxis with chloroquine was introduced in rural areas in 1975 for school children, children under five years of age, and pregnant women (Government of Zambia, 1993)

The failure of the malaria spraying program coupled with the worldwide ban on DDT adversely affected the health sector. There was need to shift to newer and more expensive insecticides in order to continue with the spraying campaign, which was not an attractive option because of poor economic growth. The failure of all spraying programs and increases in unplanned urbanization marked the beginning of the re-invasion of Zambian urban centers by malaria. Rural malaria continued to increase unabated (National Malaria Control Center, 2000).

The serious lack of resources to support the health sector caused the government to consider alternative financing mechanisms. After the Alma

Ata conference on primary health care, the Zambian government launched a pilot study to determine how the principles of Alma Ata could be adapted to Zambian conditions. The first phase of the health reforms had the following objectives:

- To respond to serious but preventable health problems in the community including malaria, diarrhea, upper respiratory infections, measles, meningitis, cholera and TB.
- To bring about the shift of emphasis from curative care to prevention and health promotion, including improved immunization coverage.

There were few successes but with slow or no progress made in many planned activities. Problems faced included little or no community participation, lack of teamwork, lack of physical infrastructure and inadequate transport.

Phase two of the reforms (1985–1990) updated the legal framework for health services, and resulted in the Health Services Act of 1985. Some elements of the Bamako Initiative were included, such as concepts of autonomy, user charges and decentralization. The first two phases were characterized by lack of coordination between the health ministry, the finance ministry, and social services providers, the result of which was poor and unsustainable health plans (Kalumba, 1991).

In 1992, a national health plan was approved, containing a new health management structure that was flexible enough to allow for private sector and NGO participation in service delivery. The plan made an effort to equalize opportunities for development in the health sector throughout the country, stressing equitable distribution of health resources to all districts facilities. The decentralized system promised financial transparency with workable accounting procedures, and with recent accounting data being made readily available on demand. The government commitment to the health reforms resulted in an increased budgetary allocation to the Ministry of Health, with its share rising from eight per cent in the 1980s to fourteen per cent in 2000 (National Malaria Control Center, 2000). Under the new plan, the government was also committed to fighting malaria. Some of the initiatives the government signed at the highest level include the African Initiative on Malaria (AIM), which has been incorporated into the Roll Back Malaria. The RBM is a global initiative against malaria, built around the principle of initiating a social movement where all sectors of society play a role in malaria prevention and control. Its main target in Zambia in the 1990s was to halve the malaria disease burden in the country by the year 2005, a goal it did not achieve.

The National Malaria Control Center (NMCC) and its partners have identified a set of key interventions that are currently being implemented at district level with emphasis being placed on districts with high morbidity and mortality from malaria. The key donor partners are World Health Organization (WHO), United States Agency for International Development (USAID)/ZIHP, United Nations Children's Fund (UNICEF) and (Japanese International Cooperation Agency (JICA).

Another possible option to malaria vector control or prevention is the use of the insecticide treated bed nets (ITNs). ITNs are a low-cost technology that poor communities can use to fight malaria. The ITNs have been found to be cost-effective in disease burden reduction, particularly in children under the age of five and pregnant women. Studies have shown that the use of ITNs is one of the tools that are very effective in malaria prevention efforts.

The ITNs are not produced in Zambia and as such their availability is quite limited. However, there is potential for the local companies to produce them, especially in an enabling macroeconomic environment of low taxes on manufacturing industries, wide markets for the product and so on. Currently, the ITNs are distributed through the public health system. The ITNs are delivered to rural health centers with the support of the district health management teams and distributed to households by "neighborhood health committees."

It is quite unfortunate that people in remote areas with low incomes cannot access the ITNs because they are only found in very few urban shops and in a few rural areas that are covered by the ITN programs. There is need to explore establishment of social welfare schemes to target groups that are unable to afford ITNs. The IEC messages developed by NMCC and its partners in the National Malaria Working Group to use in prevention and management of malaria include:

- Malaria is transmitted only by mosquito bites;
- The best way to prevent malaria is by sleeping under an insecticide-treated mosquito net every night;
- ITNs need to be treated with insecticides every 6 to 12 weeks in order to be most effective;
- Pregnant women and children under five years of age are at highest risk of serious illness and death from malaria and therefore should sleep under ITNs every night;
- Pregnant women may have serious malaria but not feel sick, which can affect the unborn children;
- As soon as onset of pregnancy occurs, women should obtain anti-malarial medicines from a health worker during antenatal visits;
- If you or your child has a fever (body hotness), you may have malaria and should seek health care immediately;
- Anti-malarials should be taken properly, adhering to correct and complete dosage (IEC materials should provide complete dosage for CQ and Fansidar); and
- If your child is taking CQ and there is no improvement within 24 hours, you should return immediately to the health center, as you may need another medicine.

6.4 Resistance to Chloroquine

Chloroquine, being the first line drug of choice for the treatment of uncomplicated malaria, is losing its clinical effectiveness as the malaria parasite in Zambia increasingly becomes resistant to it. The measurement of the clinical success of a malaria drug is classified in three categories as follows:

Early Treatment Failure (ETF)

- Development of danger signs or severe malaria from days 1 to 3 in the presence of parasitaemia;
- Auxiliary temperature equal to or greater than 37.5°C on day 2, with parasitaemia equal to or greater than the count on day 0;
- Auxiliary temperature equal to or greater than 37.5°C on day 3 in the presence of parasitaemia; and
- Parasiteamia on day 3 equal to or greater than 25% of the count on day 0.

Late Treatment Failure (LTF)

- Development of danger signs for severe malaria in the presence of parasitaemia on any day from day 4 to 14 without previously meeting any of the criteria for ETF; and
- Auxiliary temperature equal to or greater than 37.5°C in the presence of prarasiteamia on any day from day 4 to 14 without previously meeting any of the criteria for ETF.

An overall rate of treatment failure of any particular malaria drug is given by the combination of both ETF and LTF. Table 6.6 shows the current overall clinical failure rates for chloroquine for some sentinel sites in Zambia and reveals that currently, overall failure rates range from 24.1 per cent in Luapula Province (1999) to fifty two per cent in Southern Province and the Copperbelt (1997).

The implication of this is that for every four persons treated for malaria with chloroquine, one will fail to respond favorably to the drug in Luapula, while one in every two will fail to respond in Southern and Copperbelt provinces. The overall failure rates for the other sentinel sites are similarly high: Eastern Province (26.2%), Central (30.6%), North Western (34.1%), Northern Province (44%) and Lusaka (43.3%).

The four sentinel sites with chloroquine trend data available show that resistance rates in Eastern Province increased from 5.4 per cent in 1995 to 26.2 per cent in 1999, while rates in the Copperbelt increased from 28.4 per cent in 1996 to 51.9 per cent in 1997. A slight decline in rates was recorded for the other two sites: rates in Luapula declined from 33.2 per cent in 1996 to 24.1 per cent in 1999, and those in Northern declined from fifty four per cent in 1996 to forty four per cent in 1999. With reference to table 6.6, we see that the malaria case fatality has increased five-fold over the past 20 years, reflecting the high chloroquine failure rates in the four sentinel sites.

Generally, Zambian CQ resistance figures – at fifty two per cent in some sentinel sites – are lower than in some neighboring countries but considerably higher than others. Kenya and Malawi have higher resistance rates of seventy five to eighty two per cent and eighty one to eighty two per cent, respectively, while Rwanda has a CQ resistance rate of twenty four per cent. Due to the high resistance rates, all these countries have changed

Table 6.6 Chloroquine resistance patterns in sentinel sites, 1995–1999

Sentinel Sites	%			
	1995	**1996**	**1997**	**1999**
Eastern Province	–	–	–	–
Chipata District- Month	May	–	–	Nov
Early Treatment Failure	1.8	–	14.3	14.3
Late Treatment Failure	3.6	–	12.2	11.9
Total Early + Late failure	5.4	–	26.5	26.2
Adequate Clinical Response	94.5	–	71.4	73.8
Sample Size	70	–	46	49
Katete District- Month	June	–	–	–
Early Treatment Failure	5.1	–	–	–
Late Treatment Failure	8.5	–	–	–
Total Early + Late Failure	13.6	–	–	–
Adequate Clinical Response	86.4	–	–	–
Sample Sze	74	–	–	–
Lundazi District- Month	–	Feb	–	–
Early Treatment Failure	–	2.7	–	–
Late Treatment Failure	–	21.4	–	–
Total Early + Late Failure	–	24.1	–	–
Adequate Clinical Response	–	77.0	–	–
Sample Size	–	52	–	–
Luapula Province	–		–	–
Mansa District- Month	–	March	–	Nov
Early Treatment Failure	–	21.0	–	14.8
Late Treatment Failure	–	12.2	–	9.3
Total Early + Late Failure	–	33.2	–	24.1
Adequate Clinical Response	–	65.8	–	75.9
Sample Size	–	42	–	54

Continued

Table 6.6 *(continued)*

Sentinel Sites	%			
	1995	1996	1997	1999
North Western Province	–	–	–	–
Mwinilunga District- Month	–	April	–	–
Early Treatment Failure	–	14.2	–	–
Late Treatment Failure	–	19.9	–	–
Total Early + Late Failure	–	34.1	–	–
Adequate Clinical Response	–	66.1	–	–
Sample Size	–	59	–	–
Western Province	–	–	–	–
Sesheke District- Month	–	–	–	–
Early Treatment Failure	–	–	–	–
Late Treatment Failure	–	–	–	–
Total Early + Late Failure	–	–	–	–
Adequate Clinical Response	–	–	–	–
Sample Size	–	–	–	–
Copperbelt Province	–	–	–	–
Mpongwe District- Month	–	Jan	–	–
Early Treatment Failure	–	7.1	31.5	–
Late Treatment Failure	–	21.4	20.4	–
Total Early + Late Failure	–	28.4	51.9	–
Adequate Clinical Response	–	71.4	48.1	–
Sample Size	–	55	54	–
Northern Province	–	–	–	–
Isoka District	–	April	–	Nov
Early Treatment Failure	–	32.0	–	27.0
Late Treatment Failure	–	22.0	–	17.0
Total Early + Late Failure	–	54.0	–	44.0
Adequate Clinical Response	–	46.0	–	46.0

Continued

Table 6.6 *(continued)*

Sentinel Sites	%			
	1995	**1996**	**1997**	**1999**
Sample Size	–	50	–	59
Southern Province	–	–	–	–
Choma District	–	March	–	–
Early Treatment Failure	–	22.0	–	–
Late Treatment Failure	–	30.0	–	–
Total Early + Late Failure	–	52.0	–	–
Adequate Clinical Response	–	48.0	–	–
Sample Size	–	50	–	–
Central Province	–	–	–	–
Chibombo District	–	–	–	–
Early Treatment Failure	–	–	0.0	–
Late Treatment Failure	–	–	30.6	–
Total Early + Late Failure	–	–	30.6	–
Adequate Clinical Response	–	–	69.4	–
Sample Size	–	–	49	–
Lusaka Province	–	–	–	–
Chongwe District	–	March	–	–
Early Treatment Failure	–	21.7	–	–
Late Treatment Failure	–	21.7	–	–
Total Early + Late Failure	–	43.4	–	–
Adequate Clinical Response	–	56.5	–	–
Sample Size	–	46	–	–

Source: NMCC, 2000.

their national front malaria drug policies, replacing CQ with fansidar as the first line drug for uncomplicated malaria and others have already switched to artemisinin-based combination therapies or are in the process of doing so (Bloland *et al.*, 1998). Surveillance studies have shown that the change from CQ to a more effective drug saves lives and significantly reduces costs to the public health sector (Goodman, *et al.*, 2000).

The reasons for widespread resistance of malaria to chloroquine and to other anti-malarials in Zambia include:

- Treatment of clinical malaria is based on the frontline drug CQ and yet sentinel studies have revealed that CQ clinical resistances are as high as fifty two per cent;
- Erratic supply of malaria drugs to all levels of the system, namely, hospitals, health centers and community volunteers;
- Annual drug requirements are estimated to cost US$ 22 million, but Government has been able to provide US$ 6 million, while the cooperating bilateral and multilateral agencies have contributed US$ 8 million leaving a short fall of approximately US$ 8 million for drugs each year. This short fall coupled with an increasing population and incidence of malaria has led to frequently recurring shortages of malaria drugs through out the country;
- Inappropriate district planning and implementation of malaria activities based on outdated approaches to malaria prevention and control, such as residue spraying of households, cutting grass, draining stagnant water pools, clearing surrounding, etc. In recent years, however, studies have shown many of these activities to be expensive and ineffective or based on erroneous information about mosquito behavior. Districts should instead be focussing efforts on the most cost-effective interventions, such as increased household use of ITNs, early detection of fever, community-based management of simple malaria cases, referral to health centers, and effective diagnosis and malaria case management at all levels;
- High cost of treated mosquito nets and insecticides, and lack of import tax or VAT exemptions for ITNs or netting materials. Because of high taxes, there are relatively high costs of procuring bed nets and insecticides for treating nets. Until these taxes are reduced ITNs will continue to be out of reach of most Zambian households;

- The cost-sharing measures introduced in their various forms have negatively affected appropriate health care seeking behavior for malaria because access to health facilities has been greatly curtailed by the scheme. People are increasingly treating themselves with over-the-counter drugs, with no proper prescription, and with insufficient dosage causing parasites to be dormant and later to resist treatment;
- There is inadequate access to health facilities in rural areas due to the uneven distribution of these facilities. The long distances that some people have to cover in order to reach these facilities are sometimes unbearable. These geographical barriers have discouraged many from seeking health care services;
- Inadequate distribution of staff especially in the peripheral facilities in rural areas coupled with high workload has resulted in trained staff spending insufficient time consulting with their patients. Consequently, workers untrained in clinical skills take on clinical work and are thus not given time to supervise community based volunteers in malaria prevention;
- Continued focus on curative rather than preventive care has resulted in not prioritizing prevention and health promotion in community or facility levels. Policy makers have failed to put into practice the recommendations of health reforms towards preventive health care; and
- Lack of supporting supplies, equipment and printing of IEC materials, training of health workers and recurring shortages of drugs, laboratory supplies and equipment have resulted in inappropriate prevention measures, diagnosis and treatment.

6.5 Conclusions and Recommendations

It can be concluded from the material in the preceding sections of this chapter that the measures in place at present are not adequate to ensure the effective management and prevention of malaria infection in the country. In this regard, the following are the key recommendations arising from the study:

- There is an urgent need to review the drug policy with respect to the use of chloroquine as the first line treatment drug in malaria cases.

In light of the evidence on resistance to this drug and the persistently high morbidity and mortality rates due to malaria in the country, the choice of first line treatment needs to be addressed even before the authorities review other areas such as distribution mechanisms. The cost implications associated with switching from CQ to other drugs would most likely not be major because most of the alternative drugs are ready substitutes for CQ and are already available in Zambia, competing fairly freely in the pharmaceuticals market. The associated costs would therefore be mainly in terms of financing promotions to generate social interest in alternative drugs. And, considering that these alternative drugs are already available, it would be very unlikely that they will be associated with high administrative costs of adjusting. Similarly, the alternative drugs pose no major political cost because first, legislation is quite clear concerning drug procurement, and health and safety standards. Second, very little, if any, political resistance to such "switching campaigns" has been witnessed in Zambia.

- Greater emphasis should be placed on the preventive measures as opposed to the curative measures. In this regard, the government should improve access to tools such as ITNs through increasing the production and reducing the selling price. Unfortunately, according to the Strategic Plan for Rolling Back Malaria (Government of Zambia, 2000), there is as yet no national level data on ITN use. The best available data, representative of twelve districts, shows an average ITN household coverage of only 5.6 per cent. The same report (Government of Zambia, 2000) indicates that there is hope that in the future, the demand for ITNs will rise considerably to achieve a household coverage of about seventy per cent by 2010. This however is conditional on government's continued support in subsidizing ITNs and encouraging their local production on a commercial scale. Locally produced nets are reportedly supplied at fairly reasonable prices. A pilot ITN project that has been running for seven years (since 1995) has indicated that, through the re-allocation of resources from anti-malaria drugs to ITNs, the government would be able, in the medium to long term, to maintain subsidies to ITNs without encountering significant costs.
- In addition, more attention should be paid to the effectiveness of Information, Education and Communication (IEC) as a vehicle for

promoting behavioral and knowledge change. Pregnant women, children under the age of five and the chronically ill, should be particularly targeted, as they are the most vulnerable to malaria worldwide.

- Estimates show that eighty per cent of the population in Zambia lives in abject poverty. Given that malaria is a preventable disease with high socioeconomic costs, more resources should be channeled towards improving access by the populace to proper diagnostic centers, health facilities, and drugs for malaria treatment. Quick and accurate diagnoses are important in helping to generate information about the incidence of malaria in various regions. This would help policy makers to make informed decisions concerning the distribution of drugs. The need is more pronounced in the rural areas where household incomes are very low and people have to cover long distances to reach the nearest health facility. Drug distribution channels need to be reviewed to improve effective delivery of anti-malarials to peripheral health units countrywide.

References

Bloland, P.B, Kazembe, P.N., Oloo, A.J., Himonga, B., Barat, L.M., and Ruebish, T.K. (1998), "Chloroquine in Africa: Critical Assessment and Recommendations for Monitoring and Evaluating Chloroquine Therapy Efficacy in Sub-Saharan Africa", *Tropical Medicine and International Health*, 3(7):543–552.

Government of Zambia (1996), *Integrated Manual and Technical Guidelines for Frontline Health Workers*, Lusaka: Ministry of Health, Central Board of Health, Mimeo.

Government of Zambia (1998), "Major Health Trends 1976–98", *Bulletins of Health Statistics*. Lusaka: Ministry of Health, Mimeo.

Government of Zambia (1993), *National Drug Policy*, Lusaka: Ministry of Health, Mimeo.

Government of Zambia (1990), *The National Health Policies and Strategies*, Lusaka: Ministry of Health, Mimeo.

Goodman, C., *et al.*, (2000), "Economics Analysis of Malaria Control in Sub-Saharan Africa", *Global Forum for Health Research*, Mimeo.

Kalumba, K. (1991) "Towards an Equity-oriented Policy Document of Decentralization in Health Systems Under Conditions of Turbulence: The Case Study of Zambia", *Discussion Paper 6 of Forum on Health Reform*. Geneva: WHO.

National Malaria Control Center (2000), "Malaria in Zambia: Situation Analysis". Lusaka: NMCC, Zambia, March, Mimeo.

World Health Organization (WHO) (1996), *Assessment of Therapeutic Efficacy of Anti-Malarial Drugs for Uncomplicated Falciparum Malaria in Areas with Intense Transmission.* WHO Document Nō WHO/MAL/96.1077.

World Health Organization (WHO) (2001), "Zambia News Letter". *Quarterly Bulletin*, Volume 1, Lusaka.

WHO/AFRO (1999), "Framework for Developing, Implementing, and Updating Anti-malarial Drug Policy in Africa". *Liaison Bulletin of the Malaria Program*, 2(2).

Index